WOMEN, WORK AND CARE OF THE ELDERLY

We dedicate this book to:

Lloyd, Naomi, Jessica and Lewis
Kate, Rebecca and Sean

Most particularly our four daughters who
changed miraculously from little girls to young women
during the course of the research

Women, Work and Care of the Elderly

ELIZABETH A. WATSON and JANE MEARS
Department of Social Policy and Human Services
Faculty of Arts and Social Sciences
University of Western Sydney, Macarthur

Routledge
Taylor & Francis Group
LONDON AND NEW YORK

First published 1999 by Ashgate Publishing

Reissued 2018 by Routledge
2 Park Square, Milton Park, Abingdon, Oxon, OX14 4RN
52 Vanderbilt Avenue, New York, NY 10017

Routledge is an imprint of the Taylor & Francis Group, an informa business

A Library of Congress record exists under LC control number:

ISBN 13: 978-1-138-35914-7 (hbk)
ISBN 13: 978-0-429-43387-0 (ebk)

Contents

Acknowledgments

There are many people we would like to thank for the help they have given us over the last almost a decade as we worked on this research.

Our colleagues in the Department of Social Policy and Human Services at the University have been unerringly supportive of this research and retained an enthusiasm for it even when our own energies were at a low ebb and when we began to think that what we were saying must be obvious or already well known to everyone. In particular, we thank Leonie Gibbons for patiently talking through the issues, methodological and theoretical, over countless cups of coffee and tea, and Jan Mason and Michael Darcy who made valuable comments on sections of this final version of the book. To all our colleagues, heartfelt thanks for your help and support.

Several colleagues working in other universities and beyond read the original report on which this book is based and provided some particularly useful ideas for improving the final product. We thank Jill Sutton, Sharon Moore, Rebecca Albury and Robyn Munford for their criticisms and their insights. They have stimulated us and buoyed us up and kept us focused on the task.

To contact participants we relied on many people working in various agencies, hospitals, schools and universities. As we had set out to look particularly at carers working in "caring" jobs we were most dependent on our contacts in the community services sector. We wish to thank them all. We would particularly like to express our appreciation to Ian Wilson of the Wesley Mission in Sydney, whose generosity and encouragement at the beginning of the project we remember with warmth.

Our typist, Robyn Maddern, produced wonderfully accurate transcripts of the forty one interviews and did so in what were often trying circumstances. Jan Taylor, Jacqui Spencer and Marie Melvin "formatted" the camera ready copy with characteristic diligence and care.

Lastly, and most importantly, we thank our participants, the women who graciously and generously gave of their time to tell their stories and subsequently to provide "feedback" on the draft report. We hope that what we argue here will contribute to a debate about how workplaces can be changed and community services and other supports improved so that caring is made less difficult and carers' lives enhanced. We hope, as well, that for our participants this record will be an affirmation of their work and their caring and its contribution. As we say in the report, such work helps create the kind of responsible and compassionate community from which we all benefit.

The main funding for the research project on which this book is based was provided by the Commonwealth Department of Employment, Education, Education, Training and Youth Affairs under the Women's Research and Employment Initiatives Programme (WREIP). Our own institution, the University of Western Sydney, Macarthur, contributed additional funding. This enabled us to enlarge the sample and increase the number of interviews. We thank both the Department and the University for their support. The Department required the following disclaimer be included, "the views expressed in this book do not necessarily reflect the views of the Department of Employment, Education, Training and Youth Affairs."

A note on collaborative research and on this particular collaboration:

This research, and the book which has resulted from it, has been, from the very beginning, a collaborative effort. Many such collaborations have ended in acrimony or, at the very least, a distinct cooling in the relationship. This collaboration has not only survived the vicissitudes of an extremely stressful academic life in which time for research is hard won, it has enhanced our mutual respect and affection. Liz would want to put on record her admiration for Jane's wonderful sense of humour, her equability, wisdom, generosity and honesty and to note, as well, her infinite capacity for enjoyment of good food, fine wine and stimulating conversation (absolutely necessary concomitants of good research). Jane echoes Liz's tribute. Liz herself has a wonderful sense of humour, enviable wisdom, generosity and honesty. She writes beautifully, has an astute eye for detail, is a talented cook and an excellent companion. We chose our research collaborators carefully!

Elizabeth Watson and Jane Mears
Department of Social Policy and Human Services
University of Western Sydney Macarthur
Sydney
Australia

March 1999

1 Introduction

This book is about the lives of a particular group of carers. They are all Australian; in fact, most live in Sydney. They are all working carers, in the sense that they are both working in the paid workforce while, at the same time, caring for an elderly relative or relatives. The book examines this experience. We set out to explore two general questions. The first question is concerned with how the women balanced the demands of caring and paid work, how caring shaped and constrained the other areas of their lives, and the implications of this both in the immediate context of managing a stressful life day-by-day but also in the longer term. The second question concerns the kind and quality of support these working carers had received from family, community services and, most significantly, within the workplace.

The participants are all women. In concentrating on women, this study clearly recognises that caring responsibilities have always fallen more "naturally" upon women, that women are more likely to have a greater level of responsibility for care even when it is shared with partners or brothers and that they typically care for a wider range of relatives. That men may also be primary carers is important to acknowledge, but they are still a minority in the population of carers. Detailed inquiry into the special circumstances of that minority must await another study.

In taking as its dual foci paid work and family caring, our research is exploring aspects of the two main "tasks" and preoccupations of life - "the necessity to survive via some form of productive activity, whether it be hunting, gathering or working for wages; and the necessity to be social, to care for, and to be cared for by, others" (Edgar 1995, p.276). These necessities underpin all forms of social organisation. The centrality of caring both as a preoccupation - the emotional component - and as a task - the practice component - is emphasised again and again in the accounts of our participants and is a fundamental argument of this research. As Don Edgar has stated:

> *Our starting point has to be that caring is not just a burden or a problem, or a cost to private time and public revenue. Rather, it is central to the human condition and rests upon our essential inter-dependency and the inevitable*

caring about other people that arises from our close relationships with them (Ibid., p.276-7).

The words "care" and "caring" are everyday words. The term "carer" or "care-giver" is not. The use of all four terms in social policy documents and in research is relatively recent although the activity has been going on since time immemorial. That use reflects a recognition of informal caring which has been very slow to emerge. In Australia, the clearest indication of that recognition is the development of the Home and Community Care Program (HACC), implemented in 1985 as a initiative jointly funded by State and Federal governments. This very significant program set out to achieve a number of important objectives. These are succinctly summarised in the review of the Program conducted after HACC had been in operation for nearly ten years. First, it "brought the range of community care services for the aged together under a single umbrella for the first time". Secondly, it "introduced a more specific focus to community care" which had hitherto been lacking. Thirdly it "expanded the target group of these services to include people with disabilities". And finally, and most importantly for our purposes, "(I)t also recognised and provided support for the first time to those who care for frail elderly people and people with disabilities" (Standing Committee on Community Affairs 1994, p.3).

The research interest in this critical area, while it is now clearly evident, has been tardy and research coverage remains patchy. The research literature as yet provides "little local information about the prevalence of caregiving and the socio-demographic characteristics of care-givers". There is also a lack of Australian material "on the impact of care-giving on the physical and emotional wellbeing of the care-giver" (Schofield and Hermann 1993, p. 21). It is the latter deficiency which this research, like our earlier research (Watson and Mears 1989), attempts to address.

Research is always framed by important underlying assumptions and decisions about research aims, about how the research will be focused, the kinds of limitations the researchers find themselves having to accept and the strategies for "finding out" which they adopt. These determine everything that follows - the scope of the research, the data collection methods, the forms of analysis, the degree of involvement of participants and so on. We would want to emphasise four particular features of this research.

Areas of paid work investigated

The first concerns the sectors of the workforce in which we have sought our participants - the non-government (or semi-government) welfare sector and the public hospital system in the state of New South Wales. We have deliberately selected areas of work in which women predominate (in the community service sector, for example, women comprise 64.2% of the workforce) (Baxter et al. 1990, p.64) and in which the nature of the work closely parallels the task-set of the domestic sphere. The skills required are nurturing and caring skills; the personal qualities needed are those of empathy, patience and a capacity for detailed attention to the needs of others. Many of the agencies in the non-government welfare sector are church based and have traditionally not given a great deal of attention to working conditions, training or career opportunities. We were interested to see how employers in this sector had responded to the particular circumstances of our participants. It is an important and growing area of the paid workforce yet it has received little attention as such.

There are difficulties, of course, in concentrating on so narrow a range of employment settings even in a small exploratory study. In this case there was the additional risk that we might confine our participants to those who, because they had chosen this sphere of work, might also be more likely (as some would claim) to "choose" to give time and energy to caring for their relatives, rather than "choose" not to do so. For this reason we extended our sample to include public sector employees, and several from the private sector as well.

Defining what caring means

The second feature of this research we should emphasise is the very broad definition of what constitutes a major caring responsibility which we have adopted. This sets us at odds with those studies and policy initiatives which have used co-residence as the yardstick of care. Our definition has included every circumstance from co-residence to hostel or nursing home accommodation.

It has proved to be a very significant decision. Residence in a nursing home or in hostel accommodation does not mean that the carer is relieved of a major responsibility for the care of their relative. Nor is the care solely of an emotional kind. And even where that was the case, the emotional responsibilities can be time consuming and draining. You are never without anxiety concerning your mother or father, their state of health, the care they are receiving, the future.

There are very many ways in which we need to differentiate among carers and to recognise that their experiences are not all the same. The experience may vary depending on the particular disability or dependency group to which the care recipient belongs. It is also dependent on the relationship to the person who is cared for and, one might add, the quality of that relationship. In particular, where there is a history of violence, regardless of whether it is current or relates to childhood abuse, this must also have an impact on the caring experience. Factors such as ethnic, racial and cultural difference, social class and the impact of economic status, need to be taken into account in our research and in policy development and planning. But most of all we must not exclude certain people from the ambit of policy or from research, individuals who are devotedly caring for another, because our definitions fail to identify them as a "carer". When we do this, we deny their caring activity both the recognition it deserves and the material support all carers need, support which, in our view, is their right.

Policy as a lived experience

The third feature of our study reflects our particular view of the nature of social policy and should, perhaps, be elucidated here. We would want to emphasise that this is not a study of government initiatives in the area of aged care or of policies for carers. We develop an account of service provision which is based on the experience of the carers in this particular sample. Thus it is the carers' experiences, their perceptions, that form the basis for our analysis. Nevertheless, the whole range of services, facilities and programs is encompassed - community based and hospital and institutional based, provided directly through government or through private charities, volunteer or professional, Federally or State or local government funded. It includes informal support as well - family, friends, neighbours, fellow workers.

This approach to policy research underlines an important understanding of what constitutes social policy. Social policy is not just what politicians and public servants devise. Nor is it simply this together with the manner of its implementation. Social policy must always be understood to include as well, how that policy is understood and, more particularly, how it is experienced at the "grass roots". It is our view that social policy as it is conceptualised and studied should incorporate the consumer view, the client experience.

One part of the picture

The final feature of this research which we would want to underline is its limited perspective, not simply in the sense that it is a small exploratory study of the lives of a small number of women carers but, more especially, in the sense that it deals with the experience of only one half of a complex relationship - that of the carer in the caring relationship. The carer and the care recipient represent two sides of the coin, so to speak, especially in a welfare and health system such as ours in which disability or frailty generally imply informal care.

Research on carers and caring has not always reflected the significance of "the other" in the caring relationship nor attempted to explore how both parties experience that relationship. The fact that caring *is* a relationship is not always as apparent as one might expect. In part this has arisen from the context in which research attention began to be applied to the practice which we now label as "caring". This emphasis and the explicit naming of the activity was an attempt to rectify a neglect of those who did the "looking after" of dependent individuals in our society and to draw attention to the work involved. By and large the literature developed in the context of a feminist concern for the lack of recognition accorded to women's unpaid work and its importance to social and economic life.

There is another interesting shortcoming of the literature in this area. Researchers who essentially see themselves as working in the disability field have tended to neglect the experience of carers, while researchers (and others) in the caring field have tended to exclude the "cared for" from their analyses. Indeed the argument can be taken further. Much research in both "camps" appears to assume that the interests of the two groups are oppositional. As Parker points out, "feminists have tended to pose the needs of carers in ways that can be seen as in opposition to those of disabled people". On the other hand, "disabled people have asserted that they do not want care (and, therefore, do not include informal carers in their analysis)" (1993, p. 8).

There are, fortunately, some exceptions and there has been more recently a greater emphasis on the ways in which current policies in the caring field, have had the effect of "increasing divisions and conflicts of interest between [carers and disabled people] instead of encouraging alliances and solidarity" (Morris quoted in Ibid.). In addition, there have been a number of writers who have emphasised how disadvantage is something that both carers and those with a disability share. Many carers find that in attempting to respond adequately to the needs of their child, husband, wife, parent, they become themselves dependent, either on a spouse or the state.

It is important to reiterate that this research has taken as its particular focus, carers and the work they do, the sense they make of what they do and the things that hinder or help that effort. It is not primarily concerned with those receiving care, the sense *they* make of *that* experience and what enhances feelings of independence and self worth for them or what contributes to general levels of satisfaction with life and what diminishes or annihilates those feelings. Some of our participants made clear that their elderly relatives were not happy with the particular arrangements made for their care. According to the carers, some parents expressed resentment towards the carer herself, and in other instances claimed they were not in need of care or not in need of particular kinds of care or of particular services.

To state the obvious, there would not be people undertaking caring tasks, being carers, were there not other individuals who have been defined as needing care. Clearly one cannot have one without the other. But equally obviously there will not always be agreement about the need for care, either in a particular instance or, more generally, about who has the right to define others as needing to receive care.

The perspective of the frail elderly is a needed focus. As Jane Aronson argues,

> *There has been relatively little systematic enquiry into elderly women receiving care... that most research on informal care has focussed on caregivers has tended, implicitly, to objectify the elderly recipients of their care* (1990, p.63).

A study which sought to present the elderly's view of the caring relationship would uncover quite different experiences and, without a doubt, some viewpoints at odds with those of the carer. It is also likely, of course, that on some issues or in some instances, the views of carer and the person receiving care would coincide. Previous research suggests that it would also uncover significant areas of ambivalence on the part of the elderly much as has been found in relation to the experience of carers (Evers 1985, in Ibid.). Regardless of the extent of difference or agreement, a research investigation that incorporated both perspectives would be a different and more "holistic" investigation in that it would be an exploration of how both individuals involved experience "care". For this reason, it is important that we acknowledge that research that examined the perspective of the care recipient would be the complement and, some would argue, the necessary complement, of the present research.

Nevertheless, we do not want to suggest that what is presented here is incomplete and certainly not to cast doubt on the worthiness of the current research focus. After all, each individual story here constitutes a complete story and a worthy research focus in its own right. We simply want to emphasise the partial nature of all research effort and to argue that in particular cases this is of greater significance than in other cases. The argument is not just that all social research is inherently limited (that it has to accept certain in-built limitations in design), but that it can only ever present a part of a bigger picture or address only part of a larger question. The recognition of the partial nature of each piece of social research becomes particularly critical in some contexts and this is one of them.

The participants in the study

There are forty women in the sample which comprises this study.[1] They range in age from twenty two to the early sixties. The larger number were married or in a partnership; fifteen were single. This latter group all emphasised their need to continue in the paid workforce but so also did the majority of the married women and those in long standing partnerships. Most of the women held professional or managerial positions (24) or were working in a skilled trade or secretarial job (9). The remaining seven worked either as domestics in hospitals (3) or as field staff for Homecare (4), this latter group doing mainly domestic work but also some personal care work.

The periods of time for which they had been caring for an elderly relative varied greatly. Fifteen had been caring for five years or less; eleven had cared for between six and ten years; eight for eleven to fifteen years; four for sixteen to twenty years and two for twenty one to thirty years.

Mothers comprised the greatest number of dependants (19) but six of our participants were caring for fathers and six for both parents. Others cared for mothers-in-law, fathers-in-law, a grandmother, a husband and a son of a partner. One woman was caring for her own mother and father and her mother-in-law and father-in-law, all at the same time.

The elderly dependants ranged in age from sixty five to ninety five; twenty six were in the over eighty category.

We could not in so small a sample set out to reflect the ethnic diversity of multi-cultural Australia. There were, however, quite a number of participants from non-English speaking backgrounds and even more of the elderly fell into this category.

1 We actually interviewed forty one women, but one of the women did not actually fit the parameters of the study. However, she did make some interesting and relevant observations and we judged her contribution was worthy of inclusion. So although there were forty women in the sample, we drew material from forty one interviews.

Finding our participants

Most of our participants were contacted through community service agencies and regional health systems including hospitals. A few, having heard of the research, made themselves known to us or were people we already knew. Some had read about the research in an internal newsletter or memo and made contact with us; others were asked by directors or other senior staff if they were willing to participate. Those who agreed were then telephoned by one of us and an interview arranged.

Most of the interviews were conducted in the workplace, a few in the home of the participant or the workplace of the researchers. One was carried out in another university during a conference. All interviews were taped and later transcribed for detailed analysis.

The interviews were based on a relatively short list of focus questions. This allowed interviewees to provide an account that reflected their own perspective and own emphases while ensuring that, from our point of view, certain areas that we had judged to be critical to the study would be commented upon by all the participants.

Aims of the research

As set out at the beginning of this chapter, the aims of this research were twofold. The first was to explore in depth the experience of these women, looking particularly at how women balance the demands of caring and paid work, at the impact of the one upon the other, both now and in the longer term. The second aim was to examine their particular experience of services, facilities, programs and professional support of whatever kind and from whichever sector and the support or lack of it in the workplace itself.

We set out to examine the world of work and the impact of caring responsibilities on the experience of working. Our participants almost without exception wanted to talk about the experience of caring and of how stressful it was to care and work. Work might at times present real difficulties but it was the more predictable and, in essence, more manageable area of their life. The emotional toll was also much less than in their after-hours caring work. Not infrequently work was an escape from the pressures of the caring role: it was also an investment in one's own future.

Nevertheless, how employers respond to their workers who are carers is critical. And this response and its impact on employees is a major focus of this book. The book is also concerned with the effect of government provisions on the capacity to work and care. It is a fundamental argument of this research that those who work and care carry a considerable work load and that they receive insufficient recognition for this and inadequate support. This caring work saves the government, and so the community, considerable and recurring costs. If carers did not provide care then it would have to be provided by other means. Most of the alternatives are either much more costly or much less adequate or both. In their workplaces, these women are making a contribution which could not be easily replaced despite high unemployment rates and a pool of job seekers. The benefits to governments and employers are clear but the costs are great and are borne by the carers themselves. We argue that the costs need to be shared more equitably, by governments, employers and the community at large.

Caring: a conceptual morass

The social policies that address the needs of the aged, those with disabilities and their carers are clearly important to us all: almost all of us will at last become old and we could become disabled then or at any time before we reach old age. It is in all our interests that we develop good, well integrated policies in these areas. But they are also complex and contentious policy areas. They present the policy analyst with some interesting theoretical conundrums and they confront those in the public bureaucracies who would seek to develop those good well integrated policies with both conceptual and practical difficulties. These are difficulties which tend to be quite separate from the pressures to reduce public expenditure across the board or the ever present perplexities of a federal system, though both these constraints remain very much to the fore.

What confronts both researcher and bureaucrat is a conceptual morass. There are three major players or three major arenas in this policy field -

1. family and family life,
2. the workplace and labour market activity,
3. government (all three levels in the Australian context) and the issue of state responsibility.

These have been conceptualised separately and, as numerous researchers have pointed out, this has resulted in "a segmented, fractured discussion of caring" (Baines et al. 1991, p. 273). What is needed is a way of incorporating all three arenas in the analysis and a means of tracing the complex relationships between the three. This is not only an important theoretical task: it is also a significant political activity. Unpaid caring work is considered to be a private matter: how the elderly are to be cared for is regarded as something the family must resolve. Neither the state nor employers nor society at large is seen to have a major responsibility here. There is a widespread belief that caring activity should be kept apart from, and should not impinge upon, the world of paid work.

Separating work and caring

For women who work and care the experience is quite different. They cannot so easily keep the various parts of their lives in separate compartments. Nor can they separate out "relationships with elderly family members... from relationships with the labour market and state policies and programs which impact on the elderly and themselves" (McKinnon & Odynak 1991, p. 32). Writing in *Family Matters*, Peter McDonald points to the need for "future policies with a family focus... to recognise the interaction between the various spheres in the life of an individual and take account of the interactions within a family" (1993, p. 45).

Many of the participants in this study spoke of their attempts to keep separate the various spheres of their lives: none felt that they had achieved it. That such a compartmentalising of one's life should be seen as desirable, that people should feel under such pressure to keep family and paid work responsibilities separate, is noteworthy and bears further analysis. It is women most particularly (though by no means exclusively) who feel the pull between the demands of home and work, between family and career. And because it is more likely that it will be women workers who carry responsibility for a whole array of relatives, it is more typically they who experience the stress associated with juggling work and caring.

ILO Convention 156, Workers with Family Responsibilities

The context for this study is comprised of a number of elements. One of these is the International Labour Organisation Convention 156. In March 1990, Australia ratified ILO Convention 156, "Convention Concerning Equal Opportunities and Equal Treatment for Men and Women Workers: Workers with Family Responsibilities" and the Convention came into effect for Australia in March 1991. Ratification brings with it a number of obligations. Article Three of the Convention sets out the commitment to ensure that national policy is such as to enable people with family responsibilities who are employed or seeking employment to work without being subject to discrimination and, to the extent possible, without conflict between their paid work and their family responsibilities. The convention also calls for the implementation of measures which will take account of workers' family responsibilities, and do so in respect of a range of conditions and provisions, including conditions of employment, social security (Article 4), community services (Article 5(b)) and training (Article 7). This Convention, together with Recommendation No. 165, is a response to the significant changes over recent decades "in the combinations of paid work and family responsibilities which men and women are creating, in the context of wide-ranging economic, labour market, industrial, demographic and family changes". These two instruments aim "to strengthen protection for all workers with family responsibilities and to build workplaces in which men as well women have the choice and opportunity to respond to parental and other family duties" (Cass 1993, p.3). To meet its obligations the Australian Government has developed a Strategy which it launched in February 1993. This commits the government to ensuring that social, legal, educational and training provisions, employment, industrial relations and community services address the needs of workers with family responsibilities.

It is not difficult to see why this Convention and the Strategy developed as Australia's response, are critical to this research. The argument that we wish to present here is that caring for elderly relatives is an important part of the family responsibilities that many workers carry. Family responsibilities are often perceived exclusively in terms of child care. Elder care is not seen to be in the same league. If it is considered at all, it is assumed to be a caring responsibility of lesser proportions, affecting relatively few workers. Yet even a cursory glance at demographic trends suggests the need to reassess this view. If, in addition, you take, as we have, a much more wide ranging definition of what constitutes a major responsibility of care, the implication is that large numbers of people in the workforce will, for short periods or in a sustained way, be caring for their parents and perhaps other older relatives, including spouses and partners. While most older people remain is good health and are able to live independently, many will need some extra help at some time. Given the growth in the proportion of the very elderly in our community, it is inevitable that increasing numbers of workers will find themselves contributing in some way to the care of their elderly relatives. Even if they are not involved in any other way in the care of a parent or spouse, almost all will experience some degree of anxiety about the continuing wellbeing of a vulnerable elderly person. It is imperative that we do not define out of the caring equation, that constant worrying about someone whom you care about, that ever present concern for someone who has a claim upon your time and attention.

The Convention also requires that we completely reassess the taken-for-granted notion that work and family responsibilities (whatever their nature) be kept separate. This research underlines, as have so many other studies, the impossibility, the absurdity, of this mandatory requirement of the "good worker". All workers have family responsibilities even if for parts of their lives these fall lightly upon their shoulders. Yet the ideology of the separation of work and family remains very strong. The assumption is that the closer that we come to this "ideal", the more we fit the mould of the model worker, the employee who is serious about his or her work.

This a study which explores the dual worlds of work and caring and the tensions between them. It is clear that for many workers who are also caring there is guilt and stress associated with the effort to keep separate these two responsibilities and thus to meet the requirement of the good worker. Both their paid work and their caring responsibilities are important to our participants: both are important in any society.

What follows is an account of the ways in which those who work and care attempt to fit the demands of both into their lives. It is also a plea. It is a plea for greater recognition of what it is that they are doing and of how their caring enhances all our lives. It is a plea for the kind of response to that recognition which manifests itself in the form of well planned and coordinated services which are adequately funded and in workplaces that acknowledge the caring activity of their workers and support it in palpable ways.

How to read this book

This book can be read in several different ways and for different purposes. We have set out to present an account of caring that has value in the policy debate about the nature of care and about what governments, employers and the community should be doing to support carers more adequately. But books of this kind have other functions and can be of value to people who are neither policy makers nor service providers nor academics. That, certainly, is our hope.

In our attempt to capture the experience of caring and working, we have provided considerable detail and made use of extensive quotations from the interviews with our participants. We have decided on this course not so much to justify an argument of our devising but to demonstrate what complex, difficult, often frustrating and frequently poignant lives carers live and how the attempt to remain in the workforce and to continue to care complicates and heightens many aspects of caring. We have tried to take you, the reader, into this world and to set before you a picture of just what it means to engage in a continuous exercise of juggling the various demands that are an intrinsic part of it. Carers' lives are very full and demanding and so, too, in a sense, is this book.

In writing our book in this way we are aware that for some readers the sheer amount of detail will be frustrating; for others it may prove rather heavy going. We suggest that you begin with the six thumb-nail sketches in Chapter 2. These will give you some understanding of the varied lives of our participants and help make sense of the accounts in the rest of the book. In the chapters that follow, you can more easily select the amount of detail that you want to read. If you're after policy arguments then read the opening and concluding sections of each chapter and the whole of the final chapter. You can, of course, also dip into other parts of the book and savour the accounts as you choose. If you are a carer, or service provider, or general reader, you may like to read more of the detail of the actual accounts of the participants. How much detail is a matter of choice. You will not need to read every quote to understand the issues but the detail of the different situations as well as the common threads are there in the body of the book.

Detail is important in the attempt to understand the lives of carers and to appreciate their needs. The lives presented here are whole lives which are often experienced as fragmented and "stretched", as one of our respondents described the experience. We did not want to add to the sense of fragmentation. The manner in which the insights of this study have been presented is our way of honouring these women, the work they do and the contribution they make. We hope, as well, that in presenting as much of the detail as we can, it will preserve valuable material for others to use in research and in teaching.

2 Whole Lives

The women in this study have in common their participation in the paid workforce and their major caring responsibilities. The examination of this shared set of circumstances has revealed much that is common to all of them. It has also shown quite starkly how individual are the accounts and the lives that lie behind them. It is important in research of this kind, where common threads are drawn out of the whole fabric, out of the mass of data collected, that we do not lose either what is unique or, at least, different in those individual lives nor obscure the "wholeness" of those lives, the entirety of the individual experience of these different women. Each of the accounts we collected could have formed the basis for a book in its own right. We have not included life histories for each of the women, even in brief. We have, however, decided to present the reader with thumb nail sketches of six of the forty participants. These we hope will give a flavour of the variety of experiences and backgrounds and a feeling for the whole lives from which the fragments of ideas, descriptions and commentaries that comprise the bulk of the book, have been taken. In each sketch we have stuck closely to the real circumstances and only changed names and details that might identify the woman concerned.

Irene

Irene is in her early fifties and is married with three children. She lives on the South Coast, two hours from Sydney. Only one child, still at high school, remains at home. The eldest is married with children of his own and the second is still studying in Sydney. Her husband, now sixty, is a skilled tradesman and has always been self employed. At the time of interview he was having difficulty finding work and as a result there had been continuing worry about the family's income. It had been of critical importance that Irene remain in the workforce. Her wage had become of increasing significance. Cutting back on hours was not an option.

Irene, an only child, was born late in her parent's marriage when they were in their forties. Her relationship with her mother has always been troubled. Her mother was not particularly pleased to have had a child late in her life and has made that apparent to Irene from the time she was very young. Irene's father, to whom she was very close, was killed in an accident twelve years ago.

Irene's mother is the only grandparent her children have in Australia. She continues to live in her own house which is within walking distance of Irene's home. (Five years before, she had lived for a short time with her daughter after a period in hospital but it proved to be an impossible arrangement and it was the mother's decision to move back into her own home.) Her physical health is poor. She has a serious heart condition and cannot walk far because of the fluid that builds up in her legs. She has had a radical mastectomy. Her kidneys aren't functioning properly. She also suffers from Alzheimer's disease and can become very confused. She is alternately fearful and belligerent, is prone to telling lies and believes that the people around her, including her own daughter, are intent on harming her. She is manipulative, nasty and demanding and, to some extent, has been so all her life. While it is clear to Irene that she is in need of much more complete care than she has been able to obtain for her, Irene has had difficulty convincing others of this. Her mother can "turn on the charm" and appear to be relatively lucid and self sufficient for a limited period, long enough to convince a doctor that she will be fine on her own. She berates and denigrates her daughter and the care she provides on a daily basis, saying that she doesn't need care and that if she did need something done then she would ask someone else to do it.

The mother has consistently refused to accept the services that Irene has tried to arrange for her such as Meals-on-Wheels and Homecare or she has allowed them to call but not eaten the food provided.

Irene works for the local Homecare service as a field worker doing mainly domestic work. She also does the books for the family business her husband runs. Her workplace has been very understanding and given her a lot of emotional support.

Elena

Elena is twenty two and is caring for her grandmother, aged seventy one. She is single and lives in her grandmother's house. Elena was reared by her grandparents and she has a very close bond with her widowed grandmother. Her own mother lives in an outer suburb of Sydney some distance away, her aunt lives in a near-by suburb. The family are of Greek background and the grandmother speaks very little English.

Elena has been caring for her grandmother since she was about thirteen and still at school. The more intense caring responsibilities date from the period immediately after she had left school. She had just finished the School Certificate and was looking for work. Her grandmother had a stroke and Elena found herself with responsibility for looking after her. She has undertaken that care full-time until very recently when she began her first job at the age of twenty two. Since then, the caring has been fitted in around the demands of full-time work.

Her grandmother's physical health is very poor and she is highly dependent. Elena showers her and helps her with going to the toilet. She cannot be left on her own for very long. While Elena is at work she stays with the aunt or a neighbour comes in. Elena picks her up in the evening after work. She also goes to day-care one day a week. She is incontinent and this means ensuring that there is a supply of pads and washing large numbers of nappies. All the housework and general running of the house is Elena's responsibility.

Elena's job is in the private sector. It is work that involves strict deadlines and there is an expectation that people will work back on occasions. Elena cannot do that and so will bring work home when the pressure is on. Her immediate supervisor is sympathetic and supportive and this has enabled her to keep working. The senior manager is less understanding but provided deadlines are met and the business is running smoothly he makes no complaints. There is a possibility of on-the-job training provided Elena can pass the required tests.

Elena had used Homecare when she was at home caring full-time but the service was withdrawn when she started working.

Annette

Annette is in her mid fifties and cares for her parents. Annette's parents are in their late eighties. Her mother has Alzheimer's disease and severe osteoarthritis, limiting her mobility. Her father has had a number of strokes and has very poor vision. Annette describes him as "irascible". Her parents live in a house about a twenty minute drive from Annette's house. Annette does all their housework and most of the cooking. During "crisis" periods, she moves into her parents' home. Her father consistently refuses outside help.

Annette is qualified as a teacher and is also working towards a higher degree. She taught for many years, but due to her family responsibilities, resigned to take on a job where the hours were more flexible. When she resigned, she lost her superannuation coverage. She is again working full-time and has the needed flexibility but the position is a contract position. She feels her chances of completing her higher degree are considerably diminished due to the fragmented nature of her life and the fact that it is difficult to devote concerted time and energy to her studies.

Her health is not good; she feels she is eating badly and not getting enough exercise. She is tired most of the time. She finds it difficult to make time even to get badly needed dental work done.

Despite the difficulties, and the dramatic effect caring has had on her life, she felt she had gained from the experience of caring for her parents and mentioned particularly the joy she gets from her relationship with her mother.

Tina

Tina is in her late forties, is divorced and has three children, aged thirteen, sixteen and seventeen. The children are all still living at home. Tina and her two sisters share the responsibility of caring for her mother. Her mother is suffering from dementia and is in poor health. She has very bad arthritis and experiences major difficulty walking. She appears to be in constant pain but refuses to go to the doctor. Her command of English is very poor and as her health, physical and mental, has deteriorated, her ability to communicate in English has become more and more limited. Tina is very concerned about her mother. Her mother is not looking after herself and is becoming increasingly frail and frightened. She refuses to accept any community services.

Tina is her mother's guardian. She describes herself as being in a constant state of turmoil, facing daily dilemmas of when to intervene and take over aspects of her mother's life and when to pull back and preserve her mother's independence and dignity.

Tina telephones her mother every evening and spends every Sunday caring for her. She does all the shopping, washing and pays the bills. She does as much housework as she can. Her mother does not like Tina touching anything. She says she feels like a thief when trying to clean up and dispose of rubbish and rotten food. She has to sneak out with the garbage when her mother is not looking.

She works as a secretary, but would like to retrain and improve her career prospects. At present she is studying part-time at university. She gets up every morning at four to study. She would like to spend more time with her children, but there is no time. Her health is good, but she does mention that she is tired most of the time.

Karen

Karen has three children and two grandchildren. Her youngest child is twenty and still lives at home. Karen also has responsibility for the care of her parents and her parents-in-law. Her parents are in their eighties, are "getting frail" and have heart problems. Both have recently experienced falls which have resulted in loss of mobility. They live an hour's drive from Karen's home. She visits them most weekends and does the housework - cleaning, washing and ironing.

Her parents-in-law live in a "granny flat" attached to her home. They are quite dependent on Karen and this causes some stress. Their English is not good and their state of health is poor. Karen does most of their housework, as well.

Karen is the manager of a retirement village. She describes the overall management of the organisation she works for as extremely supportive and has no difficulty negotiating time off in times of crisis. She pursues the same policies with her own staff and is quick to offer support, suggestions for flexible work times and so on, if she feels her staff need this. As she argues, it is not every day of the week this flexibility is required, and so feels it is possible for an employer to be flexible. "We can cope quite wellbeing flexible when there's a need."

Maria

On separating from her husband two years ago, Maria and her three children (fifteen, eighteen and twenty three years) moved in with her mother. Her mother migrated from Europe in the early 1950s. Her English is poor and she relies on Maria to translate for her. Maria is an only child; there is no one else to care for her mother. Her mother's health has deteriorated quite dramatically in the two years Maria has been living with her. Maria is responsible for the housework, cleaning, washing and cooking for the household. Maria feels her mother is becoming more dependent and demanding.

Maria is in her mid-forties, a qualified nurse and welfare worker. She has worked as a nurse in the past and is presently employed full-time as a coordinator in an agency organising home help. She is the sole provider for herself and her children.

Maria organises her caring work around her paid work, and spends the evenings and weekends caring for her family. She gets very tired and suffers frequent headaches. She attributes the headaches to stress. Her job is stressful and her family life is stressful. She has no "leisure time". She has not had to take any time off work to care for her mother, but is confident that if a crisis arose, she would be able to negotiate time off. She mentions this specifically as a factor that to some extent alleviates her stress.

Because Maria is working full-time and living with her mother, her mother is not eligible for most community services. The expectation, Maria speculates, is that as she is working she can pay for the services that are needed. Maria's job is not well paid; she barely manages to support herself and her children; she would be unable to purchase services. As a worker and a carer, Maria has found that "there is really nothing for working carers".

A final comment

These accounts are of lives which are not merely busy, as all of us might claim our lives to be, but which are pressured, straining to fit in the myriad tasks needing to be done and coping with more than the usual emotional load - tightly "stretched" lives. We have included these brief accounts because we wanted to depict, starkly, the reality they represent and to do so in a way that underlines again that we are dealing here with whole lives, whole people, not fragmented pieces, as research of this kind may sometimes seem to suggest.

Caring is not the only activity or responsibility in these lives, it is but part of the whole. These women worked in the paid workforce, the majority had partners or were in a relationship, many had children, a few were studying; there were friends and neighbours and colleagues. But caring can and, in some instances and at particular times, did completely dominate. In all cases it shaped and was a constraint on all other activities and responsibilities. Sometimes it marred other relationships.

Whole lives can sometimes seem to be wholly taken over by caring responsibilities. Even when the caring is fitted in around paid work, there are times when it can seem to be everything, the whole picture, the whole life.

3 Where Lies the Choice?

This is a study of women in the paid workforce who happen also to be caring for an elderly relative or relatives. So it is examining a particular set of family responsibilities that it is assumed will have a major impact upon the lives of workers. The concern was thus from the beginning with two experiences, caring and paid work. Nevertheless, in our minds the work experience was seen as the starting point, not necessarily more important but the "natural" point at which to begin the analysis. Our participants, on the other hand, defined the natural starting point differently; they began with the caring experience and kept returning to it. However important work was in their lives and picture of self (and it was certainly very important for the majority of our participants), it was the experience of caring that seemed to be the most absorbing of their time and emotional and physical energy. So it was the focus of their accounts and received much more attention and was described in much more detail than the world of work. We adjusted our research lens and our methodological assumptions and have begun this analysis with the personal sphere and the business of caring.

The nature of "choice"

It is frequently said of carers, as of social actors in different spheres, that they chose to take on the caring role. Yet choice is rarely a straightforward or unproblematic thing. Not only are we constrained by the limited options "out there" in the public sphere in the form of appropriate accommodation, close at hand and with needed supports; we are constrained by the values and beliefs we hold about the proper and responsible way to behave toward those who have looked after us at another stage in our life (and theirs). Choice is rarely if ever freely made. This is not to suggest that carers are forced into caring (although a few would say that such a description is appropriate in their case). On the contrary, most of our participants would describe their "choice" as a willing one, freely accepted. Nevertheless, we would want to argue that we should use the concept with caution and recognise how restricted are the actual options available and how powerful the notions of duty of care. If a parent has an expectation that they will be cared for in a daughter's home, if they have expressed a horror of nursing homes or hostel accommodation, the "choice" is seen not to exist at all.

And having taken on caring responsibilities, many carers find that the experience leaves them with few options. If the decision has been to have the parent live with the carer, she may experience a loss of freedom to simply do as she pleases in her own home and so to make the choices that are important to most of us.

> *When I had my own place that was great. If I wanted to talk to someone, I could talk to them: if I didn't want to talk to them, I just shut myself away, read my book, played music, watched a video, whatever came to mind. But it was my choice, when I wanted to do something and when I didn't want to do something. But the choices have been taken out of my hands, that's the worst part. I'm not in control. (17)*

The histories of caring

Most of our participants, when asked to describe how it was that they have ended up with a major responsibility of care, provided a history of increasing dependency on the part of their elderly relative or relatives and as a consequence, a greater and greater involvement on their part, as carer. In some cases these histories extended over several years even decades.

> *...and all these things that had been a very gradual process and my caring had actually taken a gradual process as well. Back in 1983 she was still able to do her own housework, still able to do cooking, still able to drive. It's only in the last, say, three years that she's stopped driving a lot. Now I take her everywhere she wants to go. This has meant I am driving her here and there, driving her to doctors, driving her to friends, whatever... Late last year when the doctor found out (that she had cancer), he decided now is the time for her to have chemotherapy... She said, "Okay I'll have chemotherapy", and because of her weakened condition the doctor decided to give her a dose at home which was tablets and the lowest possible dose he could give her. It was a very traumatic time for both of us because she gave up and I was literally watching her die from day to day to day... She literally was fading away before my eyes and I'd got to the stage then, I was doing all the housework, cooking, mowing and gardening. (12)*

> *...she's been in a hostel now for over five years. Before that she was in a housing commission unit and years before, even then, I was doing her shopping her groceries and things like that, and always taking her for her*

appointments, dental appointments or buying shoes, things like that and I'm still responsible for all that today. (8)

Other histories emphasise particular crises that precipitated the need to make decisions about future care, support and accommodation.

My mother was able to live in her own unit until she was eighty one and mentally was coping fine, but the unit was three floors up without a lift and she was gradually having difficulty with the stairs, becoming more tired going up the stairs and she'd had a couple of falls while she was out shopping but she couldn't really identify why they'd happened. She'd had her name down for a retirement village for a number of years thinking that she would move into a unit and then into a hostel and then there would be nursing home care available because my husband's health wasn't the best and she felt that that would be better for her and for myself. She'd had her name down for a number of years and she'd had a couple of offers but the offers weren't ones that she was happy about and so she decided she'd wait. I think she found it difficult actually to take the final step of leaving her own unit until the summer when she was 81 and she found the heat and stairs were particularly difficult and she thought that she would need to do something. I was convinced by then that she needed to, too, because she was having occasional blackouts and I was a bit worried about her being on her own. So she agreed to looking at the hostel and she knew by then that there wasn't much point in going into a unit because she would still have the shopping and cooking. There was a vacancy in one close by here with the Baptist Homes Trust and she was given a hostel room there when she was eighty one and four months and she really settled in there quite well ...She was there for three years. She'd had a few episodes of falling in her room although she had never broken any bones, but one day she broke her hip. That was Christmas twelve months ago. She was admitted to Westmead straight away and they operated that night and there was no problem really as far as the hip was concerned. When she was in the hospital she developed a number of complications. She was getting along quite well and then she suddenly deteriorated and I thought she was going to die at that stage, she looked so dreadful, but they discovered she had a haemorrhaging ulcer and that had been triggered I think by the trauma of the surgery, so she was in intensive care for that. Then they discovered she had some heart dysfunction, which was all they called it at the time, and she was in Westmead for about six weeks and then they planned for her to go to Parramatta Hospital - there's a rehabilitation section - to see whether she'd be able to go back to the hostel or not... Anyway she went to Parramatta Hospital and she was there for six to eight weeks and they were very good in the rehabilitation section and they really persevered with

> *helping her with walking and her bodily functions were restored fairly soon, so continence came back after the surgery, it took a while. We were both very pleased about that. But the walking was much more hesitant and they took her back to the hostel and the physio and the occupational therapist went with her and they talked about whether she felt she would be able to manage and for the first week after the visit everybody was saying, yes, they thought (she could), and then they had another think and decided that it really would be too difficult for her being back in the hostel again. That was difficult because she'd really quite liked being there and she had some friends there, but it seemed the nursing home was the next step. However, there was no vacancy in the retirement village. I guess this is one of the surprises, too. You think when your name is down you just, unrealistically, think there will be a vacancy at the time when it's needed. They assured us that they would certainly keep her in mind and I could keep ringing but in the mean time it had to be somewhere else... (1)*

These accounts suggest that the "choice" to care is more usually an extended series of choices, of decisions made as the need arose. Sometimes those decisions were based on an understanding reached at some time in the past, others as the result of a gradual understanding, or acceptance, of what seemed the best, or the least "awful", of the few available options. Such decisions are rarely made without difficulty even where the available options are very limited.

> *He'd had a couple of strokes and he resisted a great deal going into a nursing home after the first stroke because he didn't want to lose his independence, obviously. I had two very young children; they were only 1 year old and then a new baby and I couldn't cope with having to turn up on the doorstep every time something went wrong. He took very ill and then went to hospital, was assessed because he was drinking very heavily as well, and they convinced him that really he would be better off in the nursing home. (40)*

A number of our participants were emphatic that the option of having their parent or parent-in-law live with them was not possible and that nursing home or hostel accommodation was the only viable choice.

> *I know my mother would much rather be with me, but I couldn't cope with her living with me. And she constantly makes little digs about it and that sort of thing... (35)*

Most of the carers who had finally settled upon a hostel or nursing home as the only real alternative had been making a considerable contribution to the care of their parent or parent-in-law prior to this move and continued to do so even though their relative's immediate physical needs might appear, now, to be taken care of by the nursing home. A number spoke of the relief in finding good nursing home accommodation especially if it was nearby.

> *I also remember how relieved I felt when we found this nursing home because the thought of (Mother-in-law) coming home which she was planning to do from the Hostel even though she was clearly not well enough. We tried two or three times to have her home again, but it was always such a stress for her and for us, it just wasn't worth it. Finding a nursing home was just a wonderful relief and I feel now that less skills are called on, that I can manage my involvement. I'm in control again basically. Which I certainly didn't feel then. (16)*

There were also stories of how some carers had felt pushed by others into decisions regarding accommodation which, with the virtue of hindsight, were probably unnecessary. Such decisions can become a source of bitter resentment and place considerable strain on the relationship between carer and aged relative, usually a mother and daughter relationship.

> *I don't have total responsibility because she is in a hostel and has been for three and a half years. She and my father moved from Melbourne to a retirement village, into a separate unit and my father died six months after they moved. I also had lost a son at the same time, almost within a couple of days of when they moved. So coping with that and their move was hard for me and then for them. Then my father died six months later and my mother just didn't cope with the total change of environment, the lack of support and friends that they'd been used to. She became quite ill and I cared for her at home for about five weeks because she refused to go to hospital (my father was a doctor, my mother was a nurse)... I found that really hard because I'm not nursing trained and I didn't know how to look after her. I took leave and cared for her at home and she did recover: I didn't think she would. That was several months after Dad died. Then the retirement village really, I felt, pushed me to make a decision to move her from the unit into the hostel and at that point in time I couldn't see her managing in the unit, so I'm afraid I opted for that decision, which I sometimes wonder whether it was really the right decision. I don't think retirement villages give people long enough to recover from illness and instead, push them into the next phase of care and for my mother who is now very well again (it does seem to have been completely unnecessary). (35)*

Those who were caring for their relatives in their own home were asked about what might lie ahead and whether there might come a time when co-resident caring and the responsibility and demand it entailed were simply unsustainable. Not surprisingly, most of these carers said that they had given a lot of thought to their own futures and their parent's. Only one was emphatic that she would never under any circumstances place her mother in a nursing home.

> *Now that she's sick I have to put her away??? No that's not the case! They (old people) are not rubbish! Even if she wasn't an Alzheimer (sufferer) and it was some other thing, I couldn't... I'd leave work, my Mother comes first... If she is bed-ridden, I can (still) look after her. I've got a big laundry there. I can make a room for her. Definitely I'll look after her until God claims her, because I couldn't live with myself. (11)*

Another woman reflected on the pain that had been caused by a decision in the past to place a grandmother in a home.

> *The doctor said when she gets too bad we'll put her into a home. But I don't want to do that because they had to put her own mother in a home and I know what it did to her. So I'm quite prepared to put up with her for as long as it takes, even though it's altered my life. I would have liked to have a family and I didn't. I'm too old now to have a family, so that's passed. (18)*

Most co-resident carers while making clear that they would care as long as they could, were quite adamant that they did not see their commitment to care as something that had no limits. If the caring responsibilities became too great, if they found that, for whatever reason, they could no longer continue to care, then they would place their relative in a nursing home. It is particularly important to note that a number of these carers said quite explicitly that it was this understanding that made it possible to go on day-by-day caring: it was not to be forever and regardless of all else.

> *I've been saving my long service leave... and I thought, well if anything happens, I'm entitled to three and a half, nearly four, months long service now, at full pay. So if I took it at half pay it would be eight months and I feel I've always gone on the assumption that between the two of us we would be able to work out how much time I was going to need with her and if she did reach the stage where she needed to go into some kind of care, that it would be obvious to both of us and she would sort of feel, okay, "Now is the time I'm prepared to go and look for some kind of care. Nursing home care". At the moment she would be assessed as eligible for hostel accommodation, but*

while I can keep her in her own home (that is what I will do). (12)

...and (the psychologist) brought up the issue of why don't you put your mother in a nursing home? But I suppose that comes back to how I feel, how I've been brought up, what's been in-built, the morals, your standards etc. and I couldn't do that to her. I personally wouldn't like to put her into a nursing home before it was necessary. I think I will know the cut off point where I'll just say it's beyond my physical endurance to be able to cope with this and you need full-time medical attention then we'll get her into a nursing home... I think Mum will know that, too. She will say, "Enough's enough". She'll either let go completely or go into a nursing home. But (at the moment) I couldn't do it to her. And, anyway, its not part of my nature to say, "Well you're in a nursing home", and then forget about her. I couldn't do that. And I'd be spending as much time at the nursing home (as I do caring at home) so I may as well stick with it. I mean I'd be feeling guilty: well she's lonely. (17)

The issue of whether or not increased caring responsibilities have had or would have implications for paid work are of critical importance in this study and are dealt with in detail in Chapter 8 of the book. What is of importance here in considering choices and the limitations upon the choices that one can make at any particular point, is how reluctantly most of our participants would have given up their paid work. Even the possibility of cutting back on the number of hours worked, held little attraction for most although others did see this option as an acceptable way out of an immediate problem. For quite a number, there was no option; they could not afford to go on a carer's pension even for a short time. And there is always the question of whether, having taken a break to care, there would really be much chance of returning to the workforce after a number of years away, especially in one's fifties.

How is the carer chosen and who chooses the carer?

The question of how it is that a particular person becomes the carer for an aged relative is clearly an important one in any study of carers and caring. In some cases there are no other possible carers, either because there is only one child and the older generation are themselves too aged, or because there may be other siblings but only one child in proximity to the elderly relative.

I suppose. I am an only child and therefore my responsibilities to my mother would be really (on my shoulders). She's the only relative I have. So I can't

> *say to another sister or someone, could you help out. If she got worse, definitely I think there would be more problems. I don't know how I'd stand as far as that's concerned. It's difficult to say. (30)*

For some it was that they were the only daughter and therefore the appropriate carer. Often there were other circumstances contributing to that solution.

> *Because I'm the only daughter. I have a brother, a delightful brother, who knows, I suppose, that I am going to assume that role by choice and also by the very structure of the family. I am older than he is and it just seems to be expected that I would be the one who has most contact. I'm also geographically closer, and then, on the other hand, I have to be fair and say that his wife's, my sister- in-law's, mother is alone too. So I think he gets caught up in a lot of helping his wife to monitor her mother who is also part of our complex and is a friend of ours too. So, if we have a family get together, all the ladies come. (33)*

In two cases the carer was a granddaughter.

> *It's because I was brought up by my grandparents from age three months. My grandmother has also got two daughters but my mother lives a bit far from here, so it's a bit difficult for her plus she's got family of her own, so she's got a lot on her plate. My aunty tries and helps as much as she can, I have to say. If I'm at work of a day time and my grandmother has got no one to come and care for her, my aunty will send one of her children up to come and pick up my grandmother and take her over there. (15)*

> *It's personality traits I think, my personality and the way I've been brought up. Ever since I can remember I was the one that did everything for everybody because I was the eldest granddaughter and it was expected. The really matriarchal type family - you never back chatted, you went to family gatherings and you did for everybody and you ran around for everybody and my nature is fairly (accommodating). I'm a pacifist and I try and to make everybody happy, whereas my sister is the opposite. My sister is very egocentric and to the point where, if she doesn't want to do it, she's not going to do it, come hell or high water. And rather than bring tempers to flare and things like that, people never bothered to ask her. (Sister) won't do it; we won't ask her. (19)*

In a number of cases the participant was married to an only son.

So, consequently, because my husband is the only son, my mother-in-law sees him as the best "fixer upperer" of her difficult problems, and legal things. And she also knows that I'm a social worker in a geriatric hospital. So I know a bit about services and things like that. (4)

Several carers pointed to the expectations of others in the family that it would be they that would carry the bulk of the caring responsibility. Sometimes that could be explained; sometimes not.

There's three daughters and one son living, but he's in Queensland. How do they see what I am doing? I've done it for so long they just accept it. They've never voiced an opinion. It just feels that I'm running myself into the ground and all they can say is, "Why don't you make him go into a home". Why can't the others pitch in and help... They are so used to me doing it. (37)

Really she's put me in charge from an early age. I'm the third eldest and it's always been me that's had to do the minding of brothers and sisters or anything like that and I really don't know why. I don't feel as though I'm her favourite. I've never felt that. So I don't really know. (18)

Some spoke of a special relationship and a particular history.

Because I've always looked after mum. I was always there. My sisters would go out: I'd always stay with Mum because she would be upset with Dad and it (was) just built on from there. We had a very close relationship. (41)

Others responded in terms of personal qualities. They had defined themselves as the carer.

I think because I do take on more myself, which I shouldn't but it's just my nature. I just can't say, "Would you like me to do it". I'll just do it. They know that we have our life and that we've got our children to look after as well and they don't like to be keeping asking us 'cause she knows that we work full-time jobs and look after our families. (23)

In several instances, siblings had contributed in the past but had been unable or unwilling to sustain that support as "the going got tougher".

Actually my sisters were a lot better then but I don't think they can cope with him now he is deteriorating whereas I'm in a situation where I see it all the time. I wouldn't say it doesn't worry me: it does worry me, but I can cope

> *with it better than what they can. (7)*

> *We both decided to bring her down with us because obviously she couldn't stay with my brother and sister-in-law. They wouldn't be able to do things for her. She was a lot more infirm in a way than she had been before she broke the hip. She was more timid. There were lots of things. So that they wouldn't be able to and, I suppose, not prepared in a way to have to do the things for Mum that she now needs doing. She wanted to go into a nursing home, but I said to her, "No". (20)*

In this last case, the carer is referring to the advantage that her nursing training (and the medical background of her husband) provided. Clearly such training is an advantage in a multitude of ways - an ability to diagnose and knowledge of how to respond to changes in the health of an aged relative, knowledge of a range of medications and their safe administration, experience in lifting patients safely and, perhaps most important of all, a capacity to distance oneself, to be objective. However, what has astounded us in this study and in our previous research is the presumption on the part of others, on the part of a family, that simply by dint of being a nurse, you are the obvious person to undertake the caring and, even more unreasonably, that a carer who is a nurse needs less support than others because...

> *You are expected to. You are the one with the answers. You are supposed to survive. You are not really a person. (10)*

Conclusion

This chapter has examined the way in which the "choice" to care is made and the way in which that caring role is then shaped by circumstances, beliefs, the availability of support from others in the family and in the community, the other caring options available, the relationship with the elderly person themselves. This has never been a straight forward matter and rarely has it involved a single or simple choice. Most caring has a history, often a long history. It has involved considerable anguish for some. It has restricted all the other choices they might seek to make in relation to every other part of their lives. The impact of the choice to care is profound.

All the participants in this study are women. It is a study of women workers who are also carers. Carers are a diverse group and include many men especially among the carers of spouses and partners and most particularly of partners who suffer from Alzheimers and other forms of dementia, from HIV related illnesses and from Multiple Sclerosis. This is not the place to examine the differences between the experience of men who care and women who care. The research did not set out to explore that territory although quite a few of our participants commented on the attitudes of men to caring responsibilities and on the greater support it was felt that men received from employers, colleagues and community services.

It remains the case, however, in our society as in most others, that the bulk of caring responsibility falls upon women. Women typically care for a greater range of relatives than men. They are more likely to be the carers of the young, of sick relatives, of dependent adult children, of the aged. They care not only for very close relatives, a parent, a child, but for more distant relatives and for in-laws as well. Quite a number of our participants had cared or were caring for several aged relatives, a parent (or parents) and a parent-in-law.

The group of carers in this study talked neither of love nor of duty in their explanations as to why they were carers although these concepts were used in some accounts of the caring experience. That the reasons for caring are not presented in terms of love or duty is not to suggest that these notions are not of great importance to this group of carers or that they did not love those they cared for. It would seem, rather, that what they were doing did not need explanation in terms of love. Typically, they provided a history of care which had nothing or very little to do with whether or not they loved or even liked their parent or parent-in-law: some commented on how little liking there was in the relationship. If there were rewards, and some were very emphatic that caring held its own very particular rewards, a catalogue of these was not produced to explain the "choice" to care. Had we asked a different question in relation to that choice and most especially if we had asked explicitly about "love" and "duty", we would, no doubt, have been presented with different ways of explaining why they were caring in the way they were. Nevertheless, it will probably always be the case that a study of this kind can only help throw light on some of the diverse factors that circumscribe and shape the choices women make in relation to caring responsibilities.

To try to answer the question of why some "choose" to care and others do not would seem to be quite inappropriate. In fact, the glib idea that there are certain kinds of people who "choose" to care and other sorts who do not, is akin to a cliche. It has seemed important to us to expose the mythology of "choice" because it is rather pervasive especially in policy circles. What has emerged from this and other research is that we struggle to care and we do so in strange, complicated and different ways. To tie our concept of care to "love" is perhaps rather dangerous simply because our notions of love and duty can tend to be rather perverse or, at least, inadequate. Love and duty are really irrelevant to "care", or their relevance is limited. Certainly these emotions or dispositions are only a part of care. The risk of sentimentalising care is an ever present one. To make this argument about the nature of care and the "choice" to care is not to take from or devalue the quality of "caring". It simply makes caring more important and much more interesting.

4 The Experience of Caring

The experience of caring has now been documented in a number of ways and in numerous accounts. Those accounts that detail the day-by-day experience of caring for a dependent adult emphasise the emotional as well as the physical load that such caring involves, whether or not the dependant lives with the carer. Almost all physical caring work involves an emotional component - compassion, empathy, distress, sadness, frustration, exasperation. Even where most of the immediate physical needs are provided for, as in nursing home care, the emotional demands of caring remain. These have been described as the demands associated with "caring about", whether or not one has the immediate responsibility of "caring for" a close relative. Caring about someone can exact a considerable toll even though and even while it may provide some of the greatest pleasures and satisfaction in life.

The emotional demands of caring

All of our participants spoke of the emotional demands that caring entails; most placed the greater emphasis on this part of the caring role.

> *(S)o with the slow deterioration we've had more emotional problems with her, basically of depression and frustration, of not being able to cope. Physical demands I've managed, you can cope. I'm very well organised, I'm independent and I can make decisions, so therefore physically, no problems. The emotional problems are the greatest (problems), Mother's constant depression and negative outlook. She's not a positive person emotionally; she's a negative person. And that is what gets me down, her negative outlook. (10)*

The emotional load was also described by some in terms of a lack of mutuality in the relationship, of having little in common, or simply of there being a limited number of things to share.

> *I guess it's the emotional side. When you're with her, there are a limited number of things to talk about in a sense. It's different if you're part of a large family and there are lots of things happening and you have different people visiting each with their different life experiences and so on... (1)*

Others spoke of the constant worry about what their elderly relative might do next.

> *Yes that's a problem, there is the worry. She hasn't gone off wandering yet, but she does do things like leave the gas burning. There's always the thought that she might do something to harm herself or the house. You don't know what you might be coming home to, what you're going to have to contend with. (9)*

The fact that the elderly parent wants to remain independent as long as possible means that there can be considerable tension associated with the carer attempting to intervene on certain important issues. Our participants spoke at length about the importance of trying to ensure that their parent retains a feeling of having as great a degree of control over their own lives as possible, but that very attempt can be emotionally draining and is often difficult to accomplish. This may be resolved in relation to the smaller things by simply letting them pass. With those issues that cannot be ignored or let rest, the problems can be very distressing. A number of accounts highlight particular instances which have involved a "wrestling" with an elderly parent to ensure that medications are taken, that financial matters are attended to. Not infrequently this has involved the expenditure of considerable emotional energy and time. Sometimes there is a successful outcome, sometimes not.

> *(R)ecently the hostel were ringing me up and they were saying my mother was refusing her medication. I'd say, "Well, I'll come around in the afternoon", and the hostel were saying, "If she has just one lot of her tablets a day; if we can just get her to take one, that's better than none", because they were worried she'd go into cardiac failure because she's having all the maintenance medication. So I used to go around there every afternoon and have this argument with this little ninety one year old lady with her hands on her hips saying, "There is nothing wrong with me, I'm fitter than you and I'm not taking these pills", and so then I'd go home crying and I'd wonder what to do and then I'd force her to take them. So then the hostel said, "Well we'll crush them and put them in her food", and they started doing that. Then they told her doctor that they were doing that and he said, "You can't do that; that's illegal". So on the Wednesday she was taken off all her medication. It was all sent back to the chemist and I didn't find out until the Thursday that they'd done that. I went straight down to the doctor*

and I said, "I'm not happy with this because she's not going to last forever but I didn't want her going into cardiac failure". So on the Friday I had to leave what I was doing here (at work), with the blessing of the OT (occupational therapist), which was wonderful, and I was allowed to go and take out guardianship for her. I had to get to the doctor; I had to wait in his surgery at lunch time; I had to get papers filled in; I had to go to the Hostel and tell them what I was doing; I had to go to the chemist and say send the medication back. I've been given legal guardianship and she's having the medication in her food. (8)

At the moment I'm going through a situation with him forgetting to pay his bills. I have to fight and argue with him. It's not for the want of money; he's got plenty of money, he get's a good pension, so the money is there... I write things on the calendar for him, write things down. His unit is being rented out he wouldn't sell the unit, he wants to hang on to that and he still wants to hang on to his car which he doesn't drive. I drive that; he gave that to me early this year. The rent gets sent to him each month and then he's got to go to the bank. Anyway, I talked him into (having) the Real Estate pay it straight into his bank. I don't want to take too much off him; I want to still let him have something to do because being in the hostel they don't have a lot to do. But it is getting a bit much for him. When I see it's getting too much for him, then I step in and advise him. He listens to me; a little bit of resistance, but he does listen to me. (7)

She had some things come from AGC (Australian Guarantee Corporation) the other day, a little bit of money, it's only a small amount, but there were documents that needed to be renewed and she'd just put them aside on the table and said, "Oh they are nothing, they are just for the tax". And I said, "Mum, let me have a look at those will you please". I looked at them and found out what they were about and then I had to tell her that they weren't for the Taxation Department, that we had to renew them and I'd have to go away and find out the best way to go about that. Don't change anything, that's what (J...) did, my father. That's the way he did it... But she's forgotten... and this is one of the big problems with her. You can't change anything, she doesn't care if she doesn't earn higher interest on her bank account. She says, "I don't care if I don't earn any interest, I just want it left as it is". So even though I think it would be in her best interest, because she hasn't got all that much money, I can't change it. I have no power of attorney, she won't give it to me; she doesn't trust me. She has nobody else to look after her. She told me one day, "I would rather give it to the next door neighbour than to you". That hurt me because I would never do anything wrong by her, I'm really only trying to do the best for her, to help her to keep going. That's one of the problems. She was inclined to draw out too

> *much money, I felt, for the needs that she has, and she's only on the pension and she doesn't have big needs, but she doesn't understand the money. So I just try to watch it and say, "Look Mum, it's very hard now; money is hard to get; they are going to change things", and... I suppose it's lying a bit... (14)*

This last account demonstrates so clearly how distressing it is to be confronted with hurtful comments and actions from someone you are trying your best to help. When the hurt is from a parent, then it is all the more upsetting. This participant, an only child, spoke of the strained relations she has, and has always had, with her mother and the anguish that has caused her.

> *It goes right the way back to when I was born... It's a terrible thing to say, but I don't think I can remember having any happy time with my mother, but I can with my father. I was just lucky that I had him. He was a very loving father. (14)*

One other carer had also to contend with constant hurtful and acrimonious remarks from the mother for whom she was caring. They were particularly common in the period when the mother first came to live with the carer.

> *As I say the first twelve months it was all pretty horrendous. There were all sorts of recriminations and generalised, nasty, hurtful remarks. I do realise that for her it must have been very distressing... My mother and I, I suppose it's fair to say, we never really liked each other all that much... Well I think the other problem is that they were married twenty five years before I was born. They had a very comfortable life and had their friends and I sort of rolled up on the scene. While I'm certain that she believes she is genuine when she says "I wanted to have a child", I get the messages, conflicting messages, "why did it have to happen to me". So there's this long standing thing... And of course now she was having to face all the stresses of the move, bereavement and the bits of dementia and all the rest of it. Those first twelve months were horrible. There were a lot of hurtful things said. And I thought I'd done rather nicely over the past twenty odd years, working through all of my reactions to what had gone before and coming to terms with our relationship. Of course that changed considerably when she had to experience living together again. So it was very unpleasant. The last two years have been progressively better and this year has been particularly good. There have only been the occasional sorts of hurtful bouts or fits of depression which are fairly reasonable in any person's life. Just to be able, in a cognitive restructuring sort of way, to say, well that's the way the lady behaves I don't really have to interpret that necessarily as particularly personal to me. That's it... There is something about my mother I dislike*

intensely and I always have done. I feel that I'm doing the best I possibly can.(9)

And another women describes her mother as someone who is very unhappy, and who "would rather die". There is considerable stress involved in dealing with her depression and her difficult and hurtful behaviour even though the carer has distanced herself from it.

She even said when she dies she's going to come back to haunt me anyway. Every breakfast we get this, "You'll be glad when I die. You can do what you like. I'm going to come back and haunt you", and things like that. And I don't need that going to work. Because I'm not a morning person anyway, and she's carrying on like that... But it doesn't worry me. (18)

Attempting to work through these kinds of difficult and hurtful relationships with an elderly parent is itself stressful. It is also very difficult to succeed. To achieve the capacity to distance oneself, as described above, to achieve any degree of equanimity, is rather rare.

I'd linger around at work as long as I possibly could and then when I couldn't possibly put it off any longer I'd get in the car and go home and I'd be howling my heart out all the way home. And I'd have to pull in down the road a bit, get myself together and go home.

And later,

I used to be somebody who was very sensitive and very caring towards the elderly but ever since Mum moved in I can really understand how people want to "granny bash". The intense flares of an anger that well up at times. (9)

Another response to emotional strain was guilt, in some cases an almost perennial feeling of guilt, and in some, resentment as well.

Yes, you feel guilty. I say, "Look, I need a night off. I need time alone". But you go out; you trudge out to Prince Henry and you cry all the way home. You think, "Jeez, I've got to do this again tomorrow". (17)

I'm feeling guilty about not being able to take her for her tests that she has to go for, especially this week. We've had to get friends up there to take her. So not being there with her. I feel a bit bad about that. Even though she doesn't expect it, though she would like us to be there. But I'm just not available to be there. (26)

There is for every carer some emotional strain associated with uncertainty about the future and what it may hold, a constant anxiety about what may happen to a parent and as a result what changes might need to be made in the life of the carer.

A sense of uncertainty, a sense of wondering whether Mother is going to - if there's a chance of her quality of life getting better. (38)

It was just after she had the stroke. The hospital was saying, there's not much more they can do for her and it was time to discharge her somewhere. We were hassling like anything to get her into a hostel where she'd get some supervision, and she was hassling like anything to go back home, thank you very much, I don't want any supervision. That was the time of some worry for all of us because we just felt she wasn't going to eat and who can we get to check on her? So that was an emotional strain - it was the worry, we were thinking of her a lot, a lot. (4)

All our participants expressed some distress concerning the increasing frailty and deteriorating health of their parent or parent-in-law. Coming to terms with that decline is never easy, sometimes impossible. Again, the emotional toll is considerable.

It does upset you to see them getting more and more frail and I've told the hostel staff that, I've told them that - I mean I go maybe twice through the week and maybe Saturday and Sunday some days and I just like to sit there and knit and Mum will doze in the chair and I'll watch the TV. I've said to them at the Hostel if I don't come sometimes, it's because I get to the roundabout at... and I think, "I've had a horrible day I can't do it tonight".

[You have to wait until you are stronger.]

Yes, I'll go tomorrow. (8)

I do understand now why. I used to criticise people for not keeping in touch with elderly people in nursing homes, but I can relate to why they don't do it now. It's just such an effort after a while to go to the nursing home to see them because they are in a place you don't want them to be and that's mentally and emotionally taxing when you actually do that. (19)

Coming to terms with failing mental capacities of someone you love and most especially, facing up to the ravages of Alzheimers and other forms of dementia, is particularly difficult and heart breaking.

> *Learning to accept the way she is was very hard... Well I don't know that I've even accepted that properly. At different times it's more pronounced than at other times. I find that very hard to accept. I see it with other people, and I can see it very clearly, but I can't see it with my own mother all the time and sometimes I don't think she's got it. But I know she has, but that's hard, just accepting the way she is and me having to handle it. (14)*

> *I think working here helps because we receive training... I really feel that has helped... I understand that she can't help it. I noticed with my husband he gets angry with her because he constantly has to tell her where things are. He thinks, "How stupid"! I don't know whether he thinks maybe she's doing it on purpose to annoy us or something, but I have explained to him that she can't help it and if you tell her something today, not only is she going to have forgotten that by tomorrow, but she's going to have forgotten something else as well. You are just going to have to come to terms with that. And I really find now I can cope with that, the fact that she asks me every night (where to put the clean dishes) when she's like that ... I know she's going to do it. I just imagine she's a visitor in this house and she doesn't know where the basins go and where the knives and forks go, so I just have to say, and sometimes I even pre-empt her question, if she's got something in her hand, I'll say that goes over there, Mum, and so I think then I don't get angry. (13)*

Not only is there emotional strain in dealing with difficulties in relationships, with the uncertainty about what the future holds and the deterioration of the elderly, the very role of carer entails enormous emotional stress. The unremitting quality of that role, the incessant demands, the constant giving out, the trying to balance all the competing demands on one's time and emotional energy, the attempt to keep everyone happy, all are significant features of the role. This group of carers emphasise them all.

> *Trying to make everybody happy. Trying to keep an even balance between satisfying all the needs of everybody else. I think in the end probably not satisfying your own needs because you feel that you were really torn apart. (40)*

> *I've got to play one thing off against another. I think most carers would find that if their person is still "with it", they would find there is this little kind of game that you've got to play. (12)*

> *Yes and that really drains you after a while because I need time out. I can't give anymore; there is nothing more to give... but you always find an extra reserve there. When that runs out I don't know. You like to believe there's always a reserve. That's the hardest, you keep giving, giving. (17)*

The histories of caring that we have collected here reveal many "ups" and "downs", crises followed by a period of relative stability, improvement followed by deterioration, but sometimes there is just one crisis after another, one painful episode, one loss and bereavement following straight on the heels of the one before. There is not time to gather strength before the next painful episode or loss. And the caring activity and the particular strains it may involve cannot be separated from the rest of one's life.

> *I find this one a little difficult to sort out given that a lot has happened in the last three years. My husband died and three months later my daughter was admitted to hospital with acute appendicitis which turned into peritonitis and I thought I was going to lose her twelve weeks later, so it took me quite a while emotionally to get over that. That was in the January and then my mother had a fall in the December and I had all of that December/January period of visiting. There just seems to have been a lot happening in the last three years. So I think it's a sort of a total picture rather than just what has happened in caring for my mother. (1)*

The impact on other family members is also an issue of concern to those who are caring in this way. Sometimes the effects have been very distressing.

> *It's on hold, everything is on hold, everything that we want to do, or I want to do, and my husband too, because he's effected as well. I can't say too much to him any more. I've been very sick and I've had lots of operations and those times that I've been in hospital, something happened that I don't know about with my mother and husband and he won't tell me what it was. But he was very hurt, very, very hurt - I've tried to find out what it is, but he won't tell me. (14)*

> *My grandfather wasn't too bad until the final stages when he was completely bed ridden and on oxygen and at the same time that caused my grandmother to regress as far as her treatment had gone. So she'd become totally dependent too. On top of that, also, my mother was a problem in dealing with it, so she was a third patient. In effect it's not just the ones you are caring for, it's the rest of the family that's involved too. (19)*

The lack of support and understanding from other family members was a source of considerable distress.

> *I just feel that they should be more supportive and it shouldn't always be on my shoulders. And it does get you down at times, it really does. (7)*

And there is simply the toll involved in doing something which makes such demands on one's time and energy, allows very little time for self and may provide few rewards.

> *Obviously I would be quite happy to be without these two major caring responsibilities. They don't do a lot for me really. The burdens I would say probably are just as strong as the pleasures. (16)*

The physical demands of caring

The physical demands of caring are, perhaps, more obvious than the emotional load: it is easier to point to what is entailed in a particular instance. Some researchers have attempted to quantify the load, to rate the level of demand involved and to calculate the amount of time that particular tasks typically consume. It is clearly important to examine these issues in ways that emphasise the sheer time demands of caring. Such calculation, such consideration of the time factor and whose time it is that is being used up, have not usually been incorporated into policy debates about caring. In a later part of this book we will examine this factor in more detail but, not surprisingly, it features here as well, as carers set out just what they do in caring for an elderly relative or relatives. But time is but one important factor and other factors are less readily quantified. When the emotional and the physical aspects are so intertwined, measuring the caring load in terms of time alone is not enough.

The physical and emotional demands are difficult to separate. The emotional state of the person cared for will almost inevitably have an impact on the way in which the care of a more physical kind is received by him or her. And both these emotional elements of the caring situation, will have a powerful effect upon the carer and make the task of caring for that person easier or more difficult. Performing acts of personal care for someone you care about, who is becoming more and more frail or confused or ill, is in itself distressing: it exacts its own emotional toll. All of these emotional impacts together with the physical demands of providing constant care, will in most cases affect the health of the carer. The state of health of the carer will determine how much physical care she can continue to give.

We have written in a previous study of " the minutiae of caring" (Watson and Mears, 1989). In the present research we were struck again by the sheer number of tasks that are performed. Some of these, such as regular telephone calls, are seemingly small enough in themselves but add them all together and the load can be seen for what it is - a constant demand, and in some instances, an unremitting load of care.

The task set that constitutes the physical side of caring is wide ranging. For any individual carer, the requirements of their own caring situation will usually constitute a subset of these diverse tasks. What each is doing is shaped by a number of factors - the level of dependency of the elderly relative, the accommodation arrangements for that relative, how close by the carer lives or works, who else is contributing to the care, the range of support from and frequency of provision of community services, and whether or not the elderly will in fact accept such services. It is also determined, in large measure, by the work demands of the carer and the attitude of employers to their employee's caring responsibilities.

The tasks that this group of carers listed included the full range of domestic tasks but especially washing and cleaning, the preparation of meals and shopping, the attending to financial and related matters on behalf of their parent or in-law, the personal care tasks such as showering, dressing and taking to the toilet, keeping a check on and administering medications and other medical procedures, taking the relative to the doctor, the hairdresser, buying clothes for her and in some cases, altering them for use in a hospital setting, and the tasks to do with social activities and outings or, more often, simply spending time with a parent and providing news and someone to talk to.

> *One of the biggest bug bears I have is paying the rent; getting to her bank account, thinking at 3.30 on Thursday afternoon, "Oh my God, it's rent day tomorrow". (8)*

> *She was totally dependent and clinging on to me. It had come to the point where she'd manage to get it (Continuous Ambulatory Peritoneal Dialysis - CAPD) done during the day but as soon as I got home, she would sort of sigh and say, "I'm not very well to-day could you do it for me". So you really couldn't say, "Well, I don't believe you". You would either have to go and prod her along and say, "Do as much as you can and I'll take over". Sometimes you could see that she definitely needed someone to do it for her. So yes, I had to play nurse. So you're doing the nursing procedure of the CAPD. You would*

also have to do the dressings and make sure the exit socket where the catheter goes in is always clean. That's quite awkward for her to do that herself. Anything else? Showering, she wouldn't shower by herself so she's totally dependent on somebody to be there, not necessarily to wash her but to be very close at hand. I'd be in the bathroom with her if she needs help. Fine, I help her in, I help her out, I help to dry her. Get her dressed, shove her neck through. It was just a general insecurity, total insecurity, real anxiety about just managing. (17)

The kind of assistance that we give my Mother, apart from the obvious emotional support, 'phoning every day and trying to visit at least once a week, the sorts of things we do are her shopping, taking her to medical appointments she is unable to get to under her own steam. She is still fairly independent within the limits of her physical disability. (29)

Since his fall I have organised Meals-on-Wheels to take meals out to him but that is only each Monday to Friday. At weekends there's a big lack. So I go out on the Saturday and do some shopping and make sure he's got food for the weekend. I change the bed clothes and put some washing on or bring it home and take it back. I clean the house, that's all done on a Saturday. Homecare come in of a Friday and do shopping. I also do his banking, he can't get back and forward to there and I've taken over his pension cheque and I take money out to make sure he's got enough money. I pay his bills as they come in. I (simply) take care of them. (37)

What I do is, I do her shopping fortnightly for her and I make little food packs, I label them and I take them over to her at the weekend and she puts them into the freezer. (16)

The importance of social activities in the lives of their elderly relatives was also emphasised. In some cases, if carers had not organised outings and visits, there would have been no real social life for these dependent elderly.

We try and make sure she has some social things happening. She takes herself out but we also try and take her out when we can. (29)

I mean I had a more sort of social support role in that sense... At the moment, because my father is in a home, his physical needs are catered for by the home and so I just provide food supplementation, fresh fruit and stuff like that. I take him out for a drive with my sister on Sunday. I did try taking my mum to see him, but she prefers to go with my sister who has a larger car and so at the moment I take my mother for a walk, I take her for the equivalent of a

> *Devonshire tea and I listen to her, obviously. So my role is basically social support, not physical. (39)*

Others placed emphasis on the monitoring role. Sometimes caring was almost solely a monitoring role; more frequently, the monitoring was built into a caring role that incorporated many other tasks as well.

> *(We) monitor that she's keeping herself warm in winter. I know that sounds silly, (but) she may not put the heater on because of the electricity bill. So, it's checking all those things. Coming to look at the flat and see that she's not neglecting herself or things around the place. Buy clothing and checking that she's wearing the right (things). We're probably overcautious but older people do tend to start to neglect themselves. (29)*

> *It really is more of a monitoring role because I'm so philosophically into them believing that they are coping and feeling independent about it. (33)*

For some carers the tasks they undertook were, at least at times, an attempt to compensate for the inadequacies of the formal services that they were supposed to be receiving, especially from nursing staff and doctors.

> *I'd just turned up at the hostel one day and he was breathing real heavy. It was a Sunday afternoon, and the doctor said, "Oh there's nothing I can do about it until tomorrow". (It was an emergency doctor). "Get his own doctor tomorrow." And I couldn't concentrate on any work that day, I kept ringing up the whole day, has the doctor been, has doctor been, and in the end I said, "I'm sorry, I've got to go because I've got to get that doctor to my Dad". I went over there and by the time they finally got the doctor and the ambulance his pulse was down to fourteen. The ambulance brought him here (hospital) and that's when he had to have the pacemaker put in. (7)*

Nearly all our participants spoke about the importance of helping the parent retain as much independence as possible. Such efforts were not without their problems.

> *She can do a bit of dusting, go out and water a few plants. Those are the sorts of things she can still do and I don't try to stop her from doing it because I feel it gives her pleasure to be able to do them. It might be hard for her to do them, but I'll tackle the things that she can't tackle. When you've got somebody who is not totally dependent on you, you can still let them do what they can and you*

kind of fit in around them. I don't want her to feel as though I'm smothering her. (12)

It's very difficult not to mollycoddle her, to let her be as independent as she can be, but then try and protect her from overdoing it, which is very frustrating. I don't want to strangle her: I don't want to frustrate her from being able to do what (she can). But then she doesn't understand her limitations sometimes, which is her undoing. It worries me, if I'm not home or I'm not around that she's up to something while I'm away, because I can't trust her. This is what she does, she knows because I don't want it, she will do it while I'm out of the house and I have to come and pick the pieces up. (10)

Emotional blackmail in not uncommon.

She says, "We've been invited next Saturday somewhere" and I might have something else organised for that Saturday and I say, "Look, I can't do that". "Oh don't worry about it, we won't go then". It's always "we". "We won't go there: you do what you want to do; just don't worry about me. I'll sit here all on my own".

[If you sent her off in a taxi, would she go, if you sent her somewhere?]

No. You have to actually take her there. I am the taxi service, the carer. I do everything. (18)

There can be other forms of resistance or attempts to control.

When my Dad got really sick I went and spent about seven to eight months with my Mum, caring for him. I was still working but I would come home at lunch time and check on them and I'd come home in the afternoon and help my Mum and often she would find that she was not able to get my Father to do certain things for her. I had just that little different way of getting around him that she didn't have and she'd say to me, "I want him to do such and such, will you see if you can get him to do it". I'd have a try and, oh yeah I'll do it for you, whereas he wouldn't do it all day for my Mum. (12)

When you are around, they don't take on the caring role. They drop it because you are there and even to the point of becoming one of the dependants while you are around. If you go for afternoon tea and coffee, everybody is there. She's been there, my grandmother has been at my mother's for a day and a half, and it will be, (carer), go and get your grandmother's pills, or put your grandmother to bed or give your grandmother a shower or a bath, even though

> *that's not my home situation, I'm out of my home, in my mother's home, and still expected, the minute I walk in the door, to be that carer. (19)*

Several of our participants described how they found themselves having to carry out some of their caring responsibility surreptitiously so as to avoid confrontations with a parent.

> *I was so busy in the physical task of looking after the house against my Father's will, surreptitiously changing sheets and washing and cleaning and washing the towels, checking Mum's underwear etc. It's easier now that I'm allowed to do it. It was when I was battling to do the absolute basic maintenance of Mum, that was the real problem. Now that I'm allowed to shower her every second night and wash her clothes and do the cooking and that sort of stuff, it's much less of a strain on me now than it was, the actual physical doing it. (31)*

Some tasks presented particular carers with a difficulty. They found them either repugnant or embarrassing.

> *When she was living with us, we were helping her (mother-in-law) a bit with eating and a bit with incontinence, but it was not as bad as it is now. I had to help her with bathing, showering and I discovered, even though I cared a lot about her, I found caring for in that personal way really difficult, particularly with someone who wasn't my own family. I found it difficult. I found a certain repugnance at some of the things I had to do, and I can remember sitting on my bed and dry retching a few times. I'm sure you've heard that from other people. It's tough: I take my hat off to paid carers. (16)*

> *I'm a bit squeamish with needles and I just can't look. Even putting her teeth back in, my husband has to do it. I just can't stand physical pain. Maybe if I'm faced with it I'll have to get used to it. (11)*

There were a number of things mentioned by our participants that were seen to make it a little easier to carry out the various caring tasks. One, already mentioned, was having acquired certain skills and knowledge in one's paid work.

> *I suppose I'm lucky I've got that bit of training behind me to look after Dad. (7)*

Another was having one's parent living near to one's own home, or near to work. If a relative is in hospital, especially for any period, then again the distance one needs to travel to visit them becomes critical.

I've clocked it, I can do Lidcombe, home, to work to Lidcombe and home again the round trip is under twenty kilometres. It takes me five minutes from work, five minutes to get home and unwind, so, I generally manage to be home at seven thirty - eight. Its a huge difference. That has taken a little bit of the pressure off and the stress in that respect. (17)

Sharing the load with other members of the family made a critical difference to a carer. We deal with this in greater detail later but it is important to note here how many were left to carry the full load of physical caring tasks on their own when there were other siblings with, supposedly, an equal concern for the wellbeing of an aged parent. In some cases a sibling was living much further away and was simply less able to perform those physical tasks. In these instances, there were some who did attempt to make whatever contribution they could and certainly made telephone calls and visits to the parent. Other siblings were rarely seen.

Only in two cases could there be said to have been an equal sharing of the load between siblings. In both cases the siblings were sisters. In one, the mother with advanced Alzheimers spent a portion of each day with one or other sister. One sister looked after her in the morning and each week night; the other sister cared for her every afternoon and for the full weekend. When one went on holiday, the other took over full-time.

In the second case, three sisters all contributed to the care of a mother who was, at the time of interview, still in her own house. She was becoming increasingly confused and fearful and so the demand on the carers had also increased. It entailed daily telephone calls from our participant, a regular Friday visit from her two sisters together, Sunday shopping and visiting from the interviewee. All gave one another emotional support and to some extent stepped in when one or other of them was under extra pressure. Even so it is difficult to share in a way that is truly equal and which attempts to take account of the different pressures on people in the other areas of their lives. The sister we interviewed tended to have to undertake any caring tasks on her own while the other two did things together. In addition she was working a full week, studying part-time and raising three children on her own. The only way to fit in study time was to get up every morning at four and work until six thirty. Finding enough time for her children, all in their teenage years, was a continual source of concern to her.

I've got only one Sunday and I wish they would come and see me while Mum is there and then I can see my sisters and my Mum all that Sunday and get it over, but because they have her on the Friday, they feel well, we've had Mum on

> *Friday. I know it is a lot but especially close to exam time, the end of semester, then I do get some support from my sisters. They will either bring her to me for a couple of hours and then they'll take her out. It's so terrible, you talk about your own mother being a parcel, a heavy load, which is quite sad. (41)*

Several of our participants commented that they did not find the actual physical load of care particularly onerous. They were well organised and physically well themselves. If they had support from formal services, could find some time to themselves and have a proper break in the form of a holiday away, then it was relatively easily managed.

> *No it's not physically tiring in that sense. Particularly now that I have home help in. I think if I was trying to fit in cleaning a house and all of those things as well (it would be more difficult). I do her washing, but that's not difficult, I just stick it in with everybody else's. I've looked after six people; I'm back to four at home plus her, so it's not in that sense all that much more difficult. You just get on with it. (21)*

But more typically, the sheer effort of trying to fit everything into already busy lives left carers feeling perennially tired and stressed. Sometimes it was hard to keep going.

> *The most difficult? I don't begrudge doing what I'm doing, let me say that from the start. The most difficult thing for me these days is gathering up the strength to do it, physical strength. And sometimes when I wake up on a Saturday morning and I'm so tired, getting myself mentally into gear to say, "Right off you go"! It's within myself that I need to get the strength to keep pushing and pushing. And I look down the track and I think, gosh... (37)*

Many felt the pull of the different areas of their lives and between the need to respond to the demands of other family members. Fitting all these separate activities and responsibilities into a day or the week increases the stress of caring.

> *At the moment my evenings are looking after my own home, having my married children come for dinner one night a week, baby sitting the baby a couple of nights a week, doing my daughter's ironing because she's got morning sickness and that sort of stuff. And the last 'x' number of weeks since my mother especially hasn't been well, we then hopped in the car Friday night and go to Blackheath and do her work and come back Sunday afternoon and put a couple of loads of washing in. And we just turn around and start again Monday morning. And in between that, I suppose some evenings I'm having my*

> *parents-in-law come upstairs for dinner or just helping them a bit, or sorting things out for them. They are very anxious people and they take a lot of time. I guess that's the stress for me because, as I said, my parents, who really have the need, and they chose to cope and my parents-in-law who don't have the physical need and yet they're under my roof and I suppose demanding my time and attention. They're very jealous when we take off, when they see their son go to Blackheath on a weekend. You know that sort of thing. But that's fine. (33)*

The importance of having a break, of taking a holiday away from the caring responsibilities can hardly be exaggerated. It was rarely a straight forward operation.

> *I thought, it's not fair on my husband and it's not fair on my daughter who was only thirteen at the time, that I have to put my mother first all the time. So I said to myself, "We are going to have a holiday". In order to do that I had to arrange it very much in advance. It was about seven months ahead. The first thing that I had to organise was getting respite care for her. I could not go away at all and leave her in the house with nobody; I wouldn't have a holiday, I wouldn't be able to enjoy it all. So the first thing I had to do was get respite care. I went to the Legacy Hostel and I booked her in for two weeks. It had to be during the school holidays because of (daughter), so she could have the holiday with us. I got that sorted out. And then, because we wanted to see Phantom of the Opera, I thought we'll have a coach trip six days and go to Bendigo Pottery and it'll be absolutely wonderful. (Husband) won't have to drive and we can all relax and just be waited on. It'll be wonderful. So I had to book the scenic coach tour to coincide with the respite care and the school holidays. I did that. Then I had to organise my own work and get my holidays approved so that I could have them at the same time. And of course, we've got our own business and usually you can manoeuvre the work around for that, so I was just hoping that we'd be able to work it out.*

> *That's what we did. But I didn't tell her. I wasn't game to tell her that I had it all organised. A few weeks before (we were to leave) I went to see her doctor, my husband and I went together, and we said, "Look, we want to have this holiday, we really need it", and he understood, of course, and he said, "Right, I'll start talking to your mother". He said, in actual fact, "I was thinking that I might have to put her in hospital", because her condition was pretty bad at the time, so he hadn't told us that before. Anyway, he went to visit her and he told her that he thought that it might be a good idea if she had some respite care because we wanted to have a holiday. Well, she told him off, he couldn't do anything about it, and then after he'd gone, we found out. She's on the 'phone to us. She went mad. She was dreadful. It was absolutely dreadful. She called me everything. How dare I think that she had to go into respite care and what*

did I think I was doing. Oh, it was just dreadful. And I said, "Look Mum, I can't have a holiday unless you do". (Husband) and I tried to explain to her that it wasn't fair on (daughter) not to be able to go away at her age. It wasn't fair for (husband) and I said, I really need to have a holiday. "Yes, all right, you need a holiday but I don't have to go into respite care". And I said, "But who will look after you"? "I look after myself. Anyway, you don't look after me". I said, "But what about all your banking, who does your shopping, who pays your bills"? "I can do that myself or I can ask (neighbour) next door. She'll do it for me". I said, "Mum, it's not (neighbour's) place and she mightn't even want to do it. She's only a neighbour; neighbours don't want that sort of responsibility when they know people are very ill. They might help you out in lots of little ways, but I don't think it's right for a neighbour to be given a responsibility like that". Well, anyway, she said, "I won't go" and she said, "That's all there is to it".

Well, before it had got to that stage I'd been telling my aunt and uncle, her brother and his wife in Sydney. They knew of the situation up here with her and they were very worried about her too. And my married son and the other son, they all knew the situation with (husband) and me. I'm sure they honestly thought we should have a holiday. So she must have got on the 'phone straight away to all these people that she knew. One of my friends who visits her regularly, I think, they must have said they thought it was a good idea. The 'phone rang next morning and she said, "Well, I've spoken to (brother) and (sister-in-law) and I've spoken to (grandson) and they all think that it would be a good idea if I go into respite care. So I'll go, but I won't enjoy myself, I won't have a good time, and don't you and (husband) ever do it again". And my husband was sixty at the time; a sixty year old man being told that, and I couldn't believe it. I've tried to be so nice and gentle with her and explain that it was going to be a really good thing for us. The Legacy Hostel is wonderful and it really is, it's a wonderful place.

Anyway, she did go and she took part in all sorts of activities. She did things that she's never done in her life before and my aunt and uncle came up especially to visit her while she was there, when I was away, and they told me later that she had a grin from ear to ear. They'd never seen her look so happy. They came away and they felt (sigh), they had this relief that she was being cared for. She won't go back, never... but she had a good time. Everyone said so, all my friends went to visit her while she was there... So that was this wonderful six day holiday that we had. But I did enjoy it. It was wonderful. (14)

Without respite, caring can be difficult to sustain. A break provides an opportunity to replenish one's physical stamina and re-establish one's emotional equilibrium. A good deal of the strain in caring is the ever present anxiety about what may happen next and how one will cope. So there is a need to feel ready in a sense to deal with whatever may eventuate, with the worst possibilities.

> *The benefits of my job are that I know all the services that are available. I'm thinking now she's in hospital, she's in intensive care, there's a sort of psychosis that goes with all of that which presents as a dementia but it may not be genuine dementia. It's the pressures and stuff of being in ICU (intensive care unit). I'm thinking, God when she finally gets on a ward, if and when, and she settles down and is back to like she was before the surgery, nothing will be necessary. But if it turns out there's a sort of post- operative dementia, which I see a lot of... then I'm going to have to start tapping into the welfare network a bit more and I can do that quickly because I know people. I just start to see if I can get some monitoring and some more help. So I'm lucky that I know what's around and what I can get. If I couldn't get into any of that then I'd have to be looking at private (services) and visiting more than I do physically. When she's well, I only need to visit once a week or so and just ring every day unless she needs me for something unusual. But if she got worse, I don't think she's going to get much worse physically at the moment, but I'm just worried about mentally. If she did get worse, then I'd have to either be able to see her more often or organise services to do that. It's hard to know in what form the extra help would come. It would be unlikely to be housework but it might be meal preparation or personal care or monitoring; I don't know. It's all hypothetical at the moment. (29)*

"And how *is* your mother?"

The state of health of the elderly relative for whom one is caring, is critical to the whole caring experience. Not only does the level of physical and emotional dependency determine the amount of support required, the increasing and severe ill health, general frailty and confusion of a close relative exacts from the carer a considerable toll. There is a great poignancy in seeing one's own parent or grandparent deteriorate and become increasingly dependent.

There are some circumstances and conditions which are particularly demanding. Dealing with someone suffering from dementia can be distressing, disturbing and exasperating. For carers confronting this reality day after day it is immensely sad. It is a circumstance of loss and therefore of grieving.

> *(W)e had three weeks at Christmas when she was in Respite again and the deterioration again has been marked since she's come home. She's reached the*

stage, even before she went in at Christmas time, I knew she'd cooked up cat food but I'd always stopped her but I went up and found her with it on the plate and in the spoon and those things started to really distress me and so that's the stage it's at now. But I guess I've reached the stage where I recognise, even say the few weeks we've been home since holidays, that I constantly am watching and I'm getting very concerned as to how I can continue to do that and be back at work. I don't think I can, so we've written to (H...) Homes with the hope that they will look at her situation and see if she can be moved up the waiting list because she's far too well to be in a hospital. Physically she's as strong as an ox and walks every where. Doesn't get lost here (at home); get's lost every where else. Mentally she's totally incapable of caring for herself. And she is often quite incoherent, her fabulous vocabulary has just completely gone and she uses nonsensical words and can't finish sentences at all. The things that she filled her life with, which were gardening and reading just aren't there. So she's still got all this energy and nothing to do with it except walk down to the shops and buy extraordinary things and come back again... (T)he only thing that gives her any pleasure is walking. So I feel that if she steps in front of a bus, that will be awful but we just have to cope with that because the only thing you could do would be lock her in the house ... Absolutely awful so there isn't an answer. She has always been very physically active, so she would probably walk three to four times a day to town and that, as I said, is the only thing that uses up her energy. (21)

A while back we had an episode where she lost two handbags, a grey one and a white one, and she couldn't find them anywhere. She searched. She's only got two rooms downstairs, one is the lounge room and one is the bedroom and just a little bathroom in the middle and a little kitchenette. So there weren't many places to search, but she had looked and I went down there and was helping her look and she got the idea in her mind that she must have come upstairs to have her dinner with us and the back door was open or something and someone had come in and stolen it. Then that fixation was there that somebody had stolen her handbag. So I said after dinner, we'll go down and turn everything out. So we turned the place upside down and we eventfully found it. She'd stuffed it some place or other, as usual. For several days after that she still seemed to come up with this thing that somebody had stolen it. (13)

(S)he needs more help, and help is available but it's her stubbornness, it's her way, it's her giving us life and that's the part that you have to deal with. It's her dignity. We could just pick her up and put her in the bath tub or we could go in forcibly and say we are going to clean your house. But it's her dignity. And that's where my sisters and I are in conflict, especially one of them. She feels she's not well and we're dealing with someone who is not well and we should

take over. But she's still your mother and you can't... That's where (my sister) feels that I'm too soft, but I feel even if she is as thick as she is, you've got to give her that respect. I went to the doctor and I spoke to him about that because I kept thinking, I am her guardian, am I really doing it properly? And he feels I'm not. He says, when someone has a mental disorder and you are going by their will, you are accepting that this disorder is acceptable. He says that's why you should pick her up and put her in the bath tub. (41)

Physical dependency can also be very distressing both for the elderly person and for their carer. To be utterly dependent on others to perform the most basic functions and at times the most personal, can be demoralising.

(M)y mother, she is very (mentally) able. She's a retired academic; she's very intellectual; she's a writer. But she's physically very dependent on other people for care. For example, she can't stir things on the stove; she can't cut bread. She told me a week or two ago she's having trouble getting her hands behind her back, so wiping her bottom is going to become a problem in the next year or two. She's very worried about that one, of course. She can barely cook, because of her hands and arms. Her rheumatologist describes her as having the worst form of arthritis he's seen. But she is very resourceful. She has a terrific social life, probably better than yours and mine. And she really has quality of life because she works at it. And that's the difference between her and my mother-in-law. (My mother) is very much a middle class, retired academic. My mother-in-law hasn't been in the paid workforce since she married fifty five years ago and her self image is of a dependent person who wants to be looked after and that's become much more so since her health has got worse. She is currently requiring help with everything. (16)

As with the effects of arthritis, the impact of a stroke can be quite devastating even when there has been a relatively good recovery.

Initially, as soon as she came out of the hospital she was with a walking frame and it took a while to get her off the walking frame and I think both physically and psychologically and she moved on to a walking stick which she still has. It's affected her ears. She's got tinnitus full-time and, as you know, it thrives on stress and my grandmother gets stressed up very easily. It's eating it's way to my grandmother's eyes too. They are slowly deteriorating and she's got the cataracts: that doesn't help either. She also got gangrene in 1987 in one of her legs, but she got operated on: luckily she's still got both her legs. She felt very helpless, like a child more or less, she felt really bad and even sometimes now she feels uncomfortable (about having to be helped with bathing and going to the toilet). But she knows that I'm there to help her and many times she says I'm so glad that you are helping me have this shower because otherwise I'd be here ten years. (15)

Dealing with the problems of heavy and binge drinking is always demanding and frustrating. The aged alcoholic or heavy drinker is no exception. The drinking simply compounds all the other problems that may be present.

If she's been drinking and she's laying on the floor, I leave her there because I can't pick her up. I leave her there and I just walk - I know it sounds off - but I walk over her and just go about my own business and then I go to bed and when she sobers up enough she'll pick herself up and go to bed. But she won't remember the next morning. And when I tell her, she says, "Ooh you make these things up to drive me crazy". I have a friend that comes over now and again too and she tells him that I do all these things to make her crazy, I'm doing it to her. He knows, because he's seen her. He's come home with me and we've found her in that situation. So I really won't have a life of my own properly until she is gone. Sometimes I wish that's soon, because I think my life is dwindling away and she's not bad enough to put into a home. (18)

Coming to terms with the deterioration in a parent is difficult for all of us. People deal with the difficulty in different ways. Some of our participants described how a sister or brother could not deal with the decline in health of their parent and so stayed away. For others the anxiety was greater if they could not see their parent more frequently and so learn to accept and adjust.

I really encouraged him (husband) to see his mum as often as he could because I think he needed time to adjust to her new condition and the more time he spent away from her, the more he would worry and manufacture things that were not real and I think the more time he spent with her, he would see what was really there and what she was really like, and hopefully be more concrete as an idea of what's happened to her. (4)

The implications of a sharp decline in the health and ability to cope of the elderly relative are an ever present worry for the carer.

But they wouldn't operate on it just in case, because she might lose the sight in her good eye. So I'm worried about the fact that if she loses her sight and becomes blind, as I've said to a few people around here, somebody who is blind can normally remember where things are. That's how they get about, isn't it. They remember that there's a chair there and this is where the kitchen is. But combined with dementia as well! (18)

Some of our participants spoke of the pleasure they received from knowing that their parent was well cared for and from seeing a real improvement in their health and general wellbeing.

> *I look at Mum and see how well she is; how clean she is; how everything about her, she just looks so much better than what she did (before she came to live with carer). She looks terrific; she really does look good. She has her bad days, obviously, but most of the time she looks good. When I used to go and visit her at my brother and sister's place, obviously they didn't notice the things, but I'd notice that, oh God, she's got an underarm smell. Well that doesn't happen any more. And she obviously looks well. She doesn't look as though she needs to go into a home. So no, she looks good. (20)*

There has developed over the years a vast literature on the behaviour problems of the young child and the adolescent and many a book for parents on how best to deal with them. There does not appear to be a comparable literature on the behaviour "disorders" of the aged, at least not an accessible or popular literature directed at helping carers to understand and to cope. The array of behaviours manifest among the aged is, no doubt, as varied as in any other age group. Most older people continue to behave much as they always have and, in a few cases, that will mean that they go on behaving in manipulative and destructive ways just as in the past. Such behaviour is not usually seen so clearly for what it is when one is young and observing the behaviour of the adults who are one's "nearest and dearest". That does not make it any easier to deal with in one's middle years. Most aged relatives do not behave quite so "badly" although there are a number of examples in this study of decidedly hurtful behaviour. What would appear to be needed is a discussion of some of the more "typical" responses to increasing vulnerability and dependency, to uncertainty and to short-term memory loss and confusion.

Organisations such as the Alzheimer's Association have set out to ensure that the public at large and carers of dementia sufferers, in particular, are made aware of the nature of the disorders and of the typical manifestations. But what is needed as well is a more general literature. In this study we can only point to some of the observations of this group of carers and the implications for them of the behaviour of their aged parents.

Two of the mothers in this study were, it would seem, particularly given to unpleasant and unreasonable behaviour and to making nasty and cutting remarks. As already mentioned, in both cases there had been a difficult and strained relationship of longstanding. There was, in both cases, dementia which was progressing fairly rapidly but in neither case could it be said to explain the "bad" behaviour.

> *There are a number of occasions particularly the first couple of years where she'd be having some sort of recriminatory stuff about no grandchildren and, I can't have friends around, what would they think and all that general sort of "whipping boy" type of stuff. Part of it, "poor me" and part of it, "It's all your fault not mine", kind of stuff. And so it would go on. And I felt increasingly, I've got to protect myself somehow from this, and, yes, she's depressed; yes, she's unhappy; yes, she would like her life the way it was thirty or forty years ago. But she can't have that; I can't give that to her; with the best will in the world, I can't give it to her. The only thing I can do is to make her as physically comfortable and give as much emotional support as I can and do the best I can. And that means I must do the best I can for me too. (9)*

Sometimes the behaviour involved others outside the immediate family and created additional stress for the carer as a result. Some of this behaviour seemed to be more directly linked to the dementia. It was not something that had characterised the past.

> *One of the things that she does is make up stories. She can tell you anything. She just makes up any sort of story. People that come in to visit her, don't know that it's made up, but I know it's made up. The neighbour opposite was very upset a couple of years ago when this happened. She made out that he was coming into the house when she was in the shower and he was walking through the house and watching her in the bathroom and all that sort of thing. And she told all the other neighbours, me included. Yes, she said, it's right and he does it to (another neighbour) next door. And I thought, oh he can't do that; he's a married man and I'm sure he wouldn't be doing that. Of course he found out about it because the other neighbours had all talked to one another and he came to my husband and me one day and he said, look I haven't done anything like that, I wouldn't dream of doing it. We knew that he wasn't, but she makes up those stories. (14)*

The self absorption of some of the elderly in this study also created problems.

> *She also, I think, really expects me to be her full-time companion and she disregards my family. Not disregards them in that she does care for them. But it's as though, why do you need to spend time with them? What about me? (35)*

(I)n that first couple of years, she went from a stage of being very demanding - all her insecurities - and very preoccupied with her own needs. Some of that came out as her sort of nastiness and demands, and a lot of it came out as pathetic, clinging, the kind of behaviour I imagine mothers would have with children they have to send off to child care centres. There are occasions she'll hold on to my sleeve as I'm going out the garage to go to work. It was initially tears streaming down the face and sobbing and the full on sort of emotional blackmail - well whether it was blackmail - she was just so desperately frightened. (9)

There were other examples of clingy and very dependent behaviour.

(T)hen he had a real setback and he won't leave the house at all. So he won't go to the front door, he won't go to the back door. He's totally dependent on me as far as that goes. He rings me all the time at work maybe two to three times a day sometimes. (37)

Resentment on the part of the elderly was also evident in some of the accounts.

(S)he can't spell properly any more; she can't add up and subtract so that when she writes a cheque I have to spell - she can spell some words or she'll start off with them all right but she'll leave letters out and I've just got to watch all the time. She didn't like me doing that, she was very antagonistic about that. (14)

Anxiety about money, losing it, having it stolen or spending it, were also recurring themes.

Her pension is basically her pocket money and she's never been better off. She does occasionally offer to pay some of the smaller household bills and then she insisted we couldn't use any appliance that used electricity. So we found ourselves having to sit in the freezing cold, (with) one bar of the radiator (on). So the utilities I pay so we can use them freely. (9)

Another concern was the withdrawal from a previous world, from former interests and pursuits, from a wider circle of friends. Not surprisingly this had an impact on those immediately around the elderly person.

She's stuck there all the time and I'd get her out and say, "Look come out, I'll take you up home". But she won't do it. She'll read, she sleeps an awful lot, an awful lot. I don't understand why she's sleeping like that all the time. If there's a mid-day movie on that she thinks she might like to see, she might turn the television on but not very often. It's changed my lifestyle heaps. I used to go sailing with my husband; we used to race. Well I don't do that any more. I can't now with mum and of course we rarely go out at night because we need to be home. And (if we do go out), I've got to cook her a meal before I go out or do something, so we rarely go out. (20)

Accommodating the elderly

This study included a wide range of caring circumstances. It incorporates not only co-residence, but the care of an elderly relative in his or her own home, in hostel accommodation and in nursing homes. This is a fundamental feature of the research. We have not assumed that the only really demanding caring activity is confined to those who live with the one they care for. A major objective of our research has been to bring to the attention of policy makers and other concerned groups and individuals the importance of that expanded definition of "a major responsibility of care" which underpins this work.

Nevertheless, this is not a study which focuses on accommodation arrangements for the elderly. And it cannot for that reason presume to make judgements about the kinds and levels of aged care provision that ought to be made available. However, as a study of the experience of caring, there is no escaping the significance for that experience of the particular arrangements that have been made in each instance for the person who is the recipient of care. Where your parent or parent-in-law lives makes all the difference to the business of caring.

Some carers in our study were confronted with accommodation arrangements that were deeply distressing to them and a source of constant anxiety. The very attempt to try and ensure that a parent can continue to live in their own home for as long as possible, can be fraught. It can place considerable physical demands on a the person "caring for" the elderly person; it can also create a heavy emotional load for anyone who "cares about" that individual and their safety and wellbeing.

Would you leave a ten year old in the house, unattended all the time? And you wouldn't, you wouldn't leave your own child and yet I'm leaving my mother in a place where she is a target to be hurt and that's what I'm facing. I keep feeling that guilt that I am the guardian, I have got that responsibility, and yet I feel well she is my mother. You take that (independent) life away from her and she won't have any will to live. (41)

In some cases, special arrangements had been made to help ensure that there was someone to attend to the immediate house keeping duties that could no longer be managed by the elderly person themselves on their own, or which they might never have had to manage.

> *So at the moment there's this lady in about her fifties. She's got her caravan there and it's just board and lodging. He's not prepared to pay anything, (but) he's very prepared to criticise, he's very critical of her. When we were there on Sunday he was just raising the roof about it. She keeps the house clean and tidy, but he wants someone to sit and talk to him all day long and he won't get that. Never ever again will he get it. He'd been married for sixty one years and suddenly that was all wiped out from underneath him and I said to him it's not going to happen again. He said, "But she can't cook", and I said, "You are never going to get anyone that will cook like Mum". So he's very unhappy, very unhappy. (5)*

In the case of co-residence, some arrangements were judged to be more acceptable than others. Where it was possible to have a degree of separation between the area occupied by the parent or parent-in-law and that used by the rest of the family, this was seen to be ideal. Needless to say, it was not always possible. Some houses were not suitable or it would have been too expensive. In other cases, the deterioration in the health of the parent had meant that it was probably unwise to attempt such an arrangement.

Where there were separate quarters for a parent there was often an emphasis on the importance of this for both parties. Being able to have time with just one's partner and children was considered vital.

> *(W)hen my grandparents lived with my parents, they were actually in a situation where it was just an ordinary house with just a lounge room and the parent was always there. In fact my mother used to say she'd have to go out for a walk. She and my father used to go out for a walk after dinner so that they could talk to each other without her being there. And I don't have to do that because we've got the granny flat; we've got that area. She gets up in the morning; she makes her own breakfast; she comes up and has lunch with us and then she goes back down in the afternoon. She usually has a little sleep. Then at night time she'll come up and help peel the vegetables or something and I let her do that, she wants to do it and sometimes I have to redo the bits that she's missed or something. Then she has dinner with us then she'll go down and watch her own television and be in her own little space and I sometimes feel that something has happened or she's done something and it's all bottled up inside, but as soon as she's gone downstairs I can say to (husband), "Oh, do you know what your*

mother just did"? and it's gone. And as soon as it's gone it's gone and it doesn't matter any more. If she was there and I had to bottle it up, it would be terrible.

And later...

But the fact that she is in her separate little domain. I think it would put a great strain on the marriage if we were in the same space and in fact I always said that would be the only condition where I would have her living with us. I can't see how people cope with having someone just sitting there all the time, listening to every conversation and everything. (13)

There must be a reason for all this

Reflections on caring, on what one gains and what are the costs in caring, are to be found at every point through our interviews. The very fact of being interviewed about their caring experience prompted review and reassessment of the ways in which that experience had shaped and constrained the lives of these carers.

Some focused upon what they had lost.

I think the greatest thing I've lost is my freedom. I think that's the greatest loss of all because I know that I can't go out at night if I feel like it. I've got to limit where I go of a weekend. I'm going on holidays and I've got a girlfriend who would love me to come away with her but there's no way my husband will go into respite care. He would get his knickers in such a knot and of course I get the silent treatment or something, it's not worth it. (25)

Others on what they had gained.

Well it's made me revalue the domestic; home work has a whole new meaning, and I mean that really sincerely.

[A valuing of what it entails.]

Yes, that's right the skill and the sensitivities. I felt that particularly with (mother-in-law)... She was a woman who in the preceding two years before she came to live with us, had lost the favoured child - her favourite son had died - her best friend had died and her husband had died and she was shattered. And helping her and seeing her regroup and pick herself up and by her eightieth or whatever it was birthday, which we ran jointly she and I, behave and be so happy and feeling so secure and well resourced and wonderful, was a real buzz. But, boy, was it hard work. I actually think that home care work ought to be paid for at industry level because it really is such demanding work in terms of planning capacity, personal skills, resilience, energy, sensitivity in particular, just meeting needs and negotiating all those demands and getting resources which really make a difference and it's a wonderful experience and I'm very glad I've had it, but I haven't actually talked about it before, so actually talking about it now is very helpful. (16)

The sheer hard work involved was stressed by most.

When we were first looking for care for her, I would have said I was spending most of my emotional energy and a lot of my time trying to organise that care and support her at the same time. I actually spent about two years, it feels like, sitting on the 'phone or visiting places, trying to get good home-based care and then good substitute care, plus supporting a woman whose behaviour was becoming increasingly erratic and doing the showering and the feeding, really hard stuff, while holding down a full-time job and looking after four children. (16)

For a few, the load of physical care had not seemed so onerous and had fitted into an already full life just as some of the existing demands were lessening. The busyness was sustained rather than noticeably increased.

Everybody's situation is probably different. I guess because we had four children fairly spread, our responsibilities have gone on longer. We have friends the same age as us whose kids have all left home and they are all (on their own) and I think, heavens, we'll be going for years yet. That's been partly our choice, too, and maybe that's been easier for me, that acquiring of (extra) responsibility. My caring responsibilities haven't really dropped enormously; I've just picked up something else along the way. It might be very difficult if you'd gone through a few years of being able to have little trips overseas and do all those things you've wanted to do and then you had to be tied right down again. I think that would be very hard. It seems to me that the responsibility to care for the aged is an area where we are not informed. Yet I don't really know that you can be informed; you just get on and deal with it. (21)

Quite a number reflected upon the way in which the additional caring responsibilities had to be fitted into lives that were already not only very full but fairly complex as well. They pointed to what they had learnt as a result of the experience. It had meant setting priorities and being organised, but it had also, clearly, required them to be philosophical about many things that it was not possible for them to change.

> *If it was just (husband) and myself I would anticipate working as I am. I don't think I'd be looking for further advancement, because I wouldn't need any more of a challenge than I've got here looking after a husband and five people, twenty four hours a day. But I would certainly consider that I'd be working full-time at least until I was fifty five, if I remain healthy, of course. At the moment it's a bit day-at-a-time sort of thing because my mother found out just a couple of weeks ago that she has an aneurism, an aortic aneurism, which means (that) any day, which could be tomorrow, it could be four years time, she's going to pop like that and she will, I suppose, just die. And so who knows what will happen then. I have always been one that family comes first and just very involved with family and I would see that settling my dad, if she were to go first, would be my priority. And so I'd have to make (those sort of choices). I guess also I'm of the old fashioned ilk that says that the home making and keeping the home going is still my responsibility, not my husband's. So I would just see that I'd have to be flexible. So it's sort of day-at-a-time stuff. Who knows. (27)*

Even the day-at-a-time stuff can become easier. This is so even when so much of the experience of caring has, seemingly, been a matter of dealing with one crisis after another and sometimes with all the crises at once.

> *The other care relationship which we have which is a bit out of the ordinary is that we've also had foster children living with us for a while. My friends and family say that I have an over-developed gene for mothering and certainly I really do like children and we had children living with us for a number of years, foster care children. I also feel we provide a sort of foster care to many other children in our community. We've had one little girl living with us in permanent care for almost four years now. The experience with my mother-in-law is particularly difficult because immediately after the stroke, when she was living with us, the week our permanent care foster daughter arrived, my husband was overseas and it was a nightmare, it was a nightmare. (Mother-in-law) almost dying with her blood pressure, almost three hundred points, me trying to nurse her and sit with her while we tried to arrange a hospital bed which took a day and this little twenty two month old, little wild animal, doing terrible things. Best not thought too much about that... It get's easier not harder. (16)*

For one or two, the experience of caring has been a completely unrewarding experience. Things have not got easier; there has been no acknowledgment of the efforts made to ensure some quality of life for the parent and no support from the rest of the family. You learn you can really only rely on your own capacities. In such circumstances you need to be able to call upon your own finely honed survival skills.

> *See even as child she's never been a mother that demonstrates her love for you; she never was one for hugging or anything like that. But you were chastised, you were belted. I was belted from an early age, we all were. You dare not get sick or anything because she would belt you first and ask why you are sick. So she was a hard mother. But now there are times when something goes wrong and you just want a hug or something or (for someone to) say, It's all right, don't worry. You never even got that. And people say, Oh, you are very hard, but that's the way I was brought up. I've had to more or less fend for myself and get by on my own mistakes myself. That's why I don't depend on anybody. I'm too independent for that reason. I don't know whether that's good or bad... I am strong enough. Maybe I was meant to be this way. I don't know. Sometimes I think there must be a reason for all this. (18)*

Conclusion

It is important in a study of workers with caring responsibilities, that the actual experience of caring is dwelt upon and explained, that it is made clear just what it means to carry a major responsibility of care. Caring transforms the life of the carer. For a few in this study the transformation was a marginal one, but for the majority it had shaped and continued to shape all activities, relationships, plans, ambitions and choices. It was a constant preoccupation; there was no shrugging off the concern or putting the worry to one side. And the physical tasks that caring entailed consumed time and energy, both in rather short supply in already busy lives.

But caring has always involved more than the time required to complete the array of tasks that are documented here. Caring is more than simply tending to the needs of someone who is dependent, or servicing other members of the household. The emotional load described here is not only the worrying about the parent or grandparent, it includes all the things that mere servicing can never provide. Our participants spoke of spending time with their parent, of listening to the account of their day, addressing their anxieties, trying in every way to make them feel as independent as possible and that they mattered and are useful and contributing. Emotional work, typically women's work, is what is being described here. This is what is entailed in the notion of caring about as distinct from caring for.

We have wanted in this chapter to highlight the fact that the caring role involves these two intertwined aspects - caring for and caring about. Policy directed at addressing the needs of carers must be based on an understanding of caring that recognises these two fundamental aspects of a complex concept, which is also a role and experience. It is also important that employers and managers are made more aware of these two dimensions of any caring responsibility. The time demands that are placed upon a carer are not just the time taken to complete particular tasks such as showering, dressing, feeding, administering medications to a dependent person, or the house cleaning, shopping, cooking, trips to the doctor's, that might help keep someone in their own home. Caring is emotional work: it is about relationships of central importance in people's lives. Caring means being with someone and attending to them: it cannot be rushed. It means worrying about them when you're not there. And when you are there, it may often mean real distress even anguish. Emotional work can exact a high toll.

In the following chapters we examine more closely the issue of time to care. We also consider the stress that caring entails and the ways in which this group of carers sought to cope with those pressures and the impact on their own health of the responsibilities that they carried.

5 Living with Stress

All the research on caring, including the accounts which we describe here, points to the stressful nature of that role. The physical demands, the running here and there and attempting to fit all that needs to be done into a limited number of hours, is stressful. But it is the emotional demands that are the most stressful of all. The impact of both on the health of the carer can be considerable. Those of our participants who would claim to be in good health physically, were quick to emphasise the emotional toll. None claimed to have survived without some cost to their health or wellbeing. And in most cases the cost was, at least at times, considerable.

The impact on health

The physical manifestations of stress are numerous. Inevitably, these are difficult to separate from the emotional outcomes. Fatigue tends to be accompanied by a proneness to being weepy or cranky or both. There are likely to be other impacts on health as well.

> *Yes, tired. Sometimes pretty miserable and cranky and therefore you take it out on the people around you. Poor diet. Tend to catch things that are very quick and easy because you don't have time to have a decent meal and also at one stage there I was getting a lot of chest type infections and colds and really run down I think... (40)*

> *Yes, tiredness is the greatest. If any body said to me, what's the major thing that you feel now, it's tiredness, but even that's not as bad as it was in the beginning. In the beginning I nearly went spare. There was a while there I couldn't bloody stop crying. Oh, and that went on not for just a couple of weeks; that went on for months. It was a pain in the neck. (25)*

Headaches and migraines are also common.

> *I've been suffering a lot from headaches. I don't know whether or not a lot of that is tension,(or) whether its a case of needing to upgrade my reading*

glasses (or) the lack of sleep and all the other things. But upgrading reading glasses requires visits (and I just don't have the time). (17)

Migraine, increased migraines. Headaches continually. Not a day goes by when I don't have headaches and a loss of concentration. It's not just the stress of my Dad; it's the stress of all the other relationships as well - husband, my children have got their own set of problems. So, yes, my own health suffers with headaches, nausea, the usual things for a burned out person just living on the edge I suppose. (37)

Sleep patterns were often affected.

I tend to take the worry to bed. And I might go to sleep for half an hour or an hour and then you wake up and your mind is going around. There are times when I don't sleep as well. He gave me a medication for that so I take that medication every night. It's not a heavy sedative; it's more a relaxing type (of drug) and it's something that you don't get hooked on. (2)

There was, in a number of instances, a tendency not to eat well; to grab things "on the run" or rely on convenience or "fast" foods. Several participants spoke of gaining weight and expressed concern about weight gain and general fitness. Others were concerned about weight loss or at least saw this as an outcome of the stress of caring. Again the emotional toll is clear.

Lack of sleep. Lack of good food, balanced food, as in sit-down-and-relax to eat it, not on the run. I've been wanting to get back into (doing some exercise). I want to loose weight and I want to get a bit healthier. Whether it be squash or going back to the gym or something like that... I just haven't had the time. So it's total lack of exercise... Smoking doesn't help. (17)

I've put on weight. I used to lose weight under stress but I've put on weight because I'm so busy eating with all these people. I eat with my Mother and I eat with my Father. In some ways I'm looking after myself a bit better because I'm so terrified about getting cancer myself now. I am trying to rest. (36)

I lose a lot of weight when he's in hospital. I find that my eating patterns are poor. Yes, just being generally run down. (22)

Problems with lower back pain feature in all our research on carers.

I suffer from a bad back. I have had to do lifting, like help Mum up out of the lounge. I learnt through one bad experience from sort of bending over and I thought, "Bend your knees, girl, bend your knees". So I know how to do it. But sometimes you don't think. (17)

Hernias are another recurring ailment also clearly linked with lifting and other straining activity.

I also suffer with arthritis, and I'm on (medication) and I've got two hernias. I've got a hiatus hernia and a tummy one, so I'm on (medication) for those as well. And I can't really work much more than what I'm doing. (14)

Being vulnerable to infections of every kind is a not surprising manifestation of stress.

I've never even thought of this. The last five years, it's maybe also sort of ageing, but I've been much more vulnerable to viruses, to colds, to sleepless nights, range of mild stress-related minor ailments than I ever was before. So, yes, probably. But I can actually switch off fairly easily and recoup quite quickly. (16)

Existing conditions were exacerbated by the stress of caring.

I have asthma and I did have a very bad attack of asthma but that was when Mum was very sick. She'd just gotten over an operation and that's when it always happens, when suddenly you can stop. (32)

Quite a few of the carers in this study judged their physical health to be good, indeed, very good in some cases. To be in good health is an enormous advantage when taking on a stressful caring load.

No, I'm fairly healthy. (7)

The emotional or psychological manifestations of stress have already been alluded to. For most of these carers they were the effects that they were most aware of and which they found particularly distressing.

Health? Anxiety! I was down in a very bad depression for about six or eight months. I'm not saying it's just that. Probably a little bit of everything. Getting married young, bringing up children very young and working at the same time, plus, trying to look after your parents and trying not to let them know that your husband gets upset because you're helping your parents. (23)

A number spoke of being "up tight" or "on a short fuse".

Yes I think they (caring responsibilities) make me quite stressed. You are fairly constantly uptight because you've got that feeling that you can't relax. (35)

And most graphically!

I had reached the point where I did need to take some kind of action because I was like a short fuse about to be lit. Like a volcano and I was capping the top of the volcano all the time and as I said to my boss, sometimes I feel like a volcano is inside me and every time I get stressed, I'm putting a plug in the top of the volcano to stop it exploding. One of these days I'm going to cap that, put a plug in the top of it and it's just going to explode out the side like Mt. St. Helens. So I had to find a way of being able to defuse that by syphoning it off from the bottom. I work very much in mental pictures. (12)

The nature of the stress of caring

The concept of stress has become a commonplace notion in contemporary life. Nevertheless, pinpointing just precisely what it is, what the term means, still poses some difficulties. It is easier to describe the manifestations, as above, and even to isolate causes, than to pin down what it is that we are dealing with. This chapter is not a treatise on the nature of stress. We do not have the competence to enter upon that particular discourse. Nor is stress, as a phenomenon, a primary focus of the study. But what we can provide here are the insights which our participants offered of their own experience of stress as they shouldered a major responsibility of care for an aged relative.

For some stress was experienced as a constant pressure or demand, an ever present sense of being responsible for others and their welfare, of not being able to "let go".

It's that fact that I'm always conscious that there's a responsibility there, that I couldn't possibly go and be frivolous and irresponsible. I'm not that by nature anyway, but there isn't the room for that. And I look at the young ones on the staff and off they go to do their own thing and I think, "Good heavens, fancy doing that". It's a long time since I have been able to, and I don't know that I want to, it's just that recognition that my lifestyle is quite different. (21)

...the lack of freedom to devote time to my children, not to be able to spontaneously go and do something with them because I've got to see that Mother's fed; I've got to see that Mother's taken care of. So, therefore, I just can't dump things. I notice the difference when she's hospitalised. Just how, it takes me a week to pick back up. I feel totally run down as soon as I get her hospitalised. I'm just starting to feel more comfortable after about a week. So obviously it does wear me down emotionally. But I don't give in and it hasn't affected me to the point of nervous exhaustion, but I obviously must experience it because I just notice when she's hospitalised or my brother takes her for a week, the difference I feel. Or if I go away, I don't want to come back. I don't feel like being harnessed again, but then you do... Yes, I have suffered episodes of nervous exhaustion. Yes, I think it has been the extra pressures. (10)

The dual, work and caring, the stresses? Oh they're enormous. You have to prioritise every day and say, what is your priority? You have to play your priority, be it work, be it your husband, be it your family. And, again, it's just that guilt, the guilt that runs through all the time and it just sits with me and I have a lot of trouble with that. (22)

Just that constant sense of responsibility. I think you tend to think that as your children are getting older you are going to step out of that sense that you have when you've got little children, of never being able to just switch off for a moment from your responsibility and I guess you are going into a period in your life where you think you are going to be free from responsibility and instead you are becoming more and more responsible for someone who is not capable of learning, (whereas) with a child... I guess the fact that one is always organised and you just occasionally want to be disorganised. Just that sense that there is no room within that to just be frivolous. I can't imagine being frivolous. To do something impulsive would be out of the question. Maybe I'm not an impulsive person, I don't know, but I certainly would not have the capacity to find that out at this stage. We couldn't say let's drop everything and go to... that doesn't matter, but there is that sense and I cope with it quite well because I've got a lot of support. I would think for some people... it would drive them mad, I think, because that would end up being all you could see, the fact that never, never did you have a life of your own to any extent at all. Our circumstance is such that it doesn't get to be disproportionately awful. I would say that's the most difficult thing, just that sense of constant responsibility. But I think women carry that any way and I don't know that we are terribly good at letting go of it when our children get bigger anyway. (21)

Some of our participants spoke of stress being experienced as an emotional load, as uncertainty and even dread about the future, as a sense of poignancy or as distress. Guilt also features here as elsewhere in the accounts.

> *I don't think the stress of caring, just the stress of having an aged Mother whose health might deteriorate or she may die at any time because of the illnesses she's got. That stress is there all the time. That's why I ring everyday and worry if she doesn't answer the 'phone. I need to monitor that for my own peace of mind. (29)*

> *But I don't know how much longer that's going to go on (i.e., mother managing in her own house) and what I have not faced. I don't know; I haven't gone that far. I know that it will happen. Another thing that struck me was that I'm the only one that's looking after her. I was sick a couple of months ago and I had to stay in bed a few days and I suddenly thought, it sounds terrible, but, what would happen if I died and what would happen to her? (14)*

> *I think it can be quite depressing because you are watching deterioration. (5)*

As is clear in the accounts above, the relationship with the person for whom you are caring can itself be a source of stress. In most cases a new relationship is having to be worked out. There are many cases where carers experienced a role reversal and some difficulties in that new circumstance. The daughter may feel she has in a sense become the mother, but it is never quite that straightforward. One's mother doesn't cease to be one's mother even if her behaviour has become childlike due to dementia.

> *Very much the fact that as long as they haven't got dementia, the person that you are dealing with is not a child. But they are dependent and you literally have to learn how to handle them as an adult rather than treating them as a child, because they are an adult. If they've got dementia to a certain extent you can treat them as a child, but when they are fully compos mentis you have to be very aware and that's a stressful thing in itself. Because they are adult and have all their faculties and own ideas about what they want and expect and consequently you had to take that into consideration or find ways to manoeuvre around it. And you have to take into consideration the fact that you don't want the person to feel that you are taking over. (12)*

In some cases, the relationships were particularly difficult. We have already described several cases where the relationship between mother and daughter had always been strained. There were other instances where the quality of the relationship was less distressing but nevertheless stressful. This was so for a range of reasons. In one case it was a mother used to getting her own way, used to being the one who makes all the decisions, who is always right.

> *I've had experience because I've done nursing, psychiatric nursing. That helps. But living with an elderly person you know that they're set in their ways, that they're difficult to change. There's also three generations living there, so they've got a lot of family problems. Because she's the matriarch, she expects things done her way and although she's trying to be a little bit more tolerant, there's a lot of problems emotionally. So it's not just physical problems, but there are a lot of emotional problems. Because I've got a lady who's used to having her own way, who believes whatever she says is right, being an ethnic background as well. (30)*

In another instance, the carer spoke of the tremendous strain that had been involved in taking on the care of her father after her mother's death. That loss was traumatic enough but in addition she had found herself with a father who was becoming increasingly dependent and demanding. She was having to draw back from the relationship and assert her own need for time apart and a degree of detachment. That too has been stressful.

> *Just knowing that he's there (in his own home) and not being sufficiently well cared for is a very great stress within itself without constantly being given these other things to do. Because with every little job you plan beforehand and it all requires steps that its just further stress on your day. To cope again, sometimes I feel I have to step back, which is dreadful, but I'm finding that I'm stepping back more and more just so that I can try and look from a distance and not become too drawn in. Sometimes I need the odd weekend away but I give him a ring and see that he's okay. I'm not making the twice weekly visits; I'm trying to go a week without calling in and he's starting to accept that now. But then when he does see me he makes comments like, "Hello stranger", or, "I know that I'm a burden to you", and things like that which tug at you even more. I feel in the last two to two and a half years that it has got on top of me. I really think I've aged considerably... It's the emotional demands that are greatest. Losing my mother was very traumatic; it was very hard for me and then to have to look after him in that capacity, because I then had to step into her caring role and because the way it affected him was that his health worsened and emotionally he didn't cope very well at all that I then went straight into a very deep caring role for him. And* ***my*** *health was breaking down (as well), so that didn't help things at all there. (22)*

Where one is caring for both one's parents it can be difficult to negotiate a caring arrangement that is a realistic one, one that reflects the level of dependency, of need, that each parent has. One parent refused to accept the extent of decline in their partner and thus to allow the daughter to provide the care that is needed. The stress that this has created has been acute.

> *My main problem has been to get him to recognise the situation that my mother is in. The situation is a fluid one, a changing one. The problem started to escalate rapidly in 1990, but the crisis period was really from 1990 to April this year when I could not get past him to get my mother to a doctor, except for one acute period when she was hospitalised because of a severe internal bleed. (This was because of) wrong medication which I had illegally got a doctor to slip to me because I couldn't get her to a doctor to get it properly assessed. My father is now allowing her to see a doctor and he's at least allowing the Sydney Home Nursing Service nurse in once a week, but he won't allow her to do anything. She's just trying to find an excuse to keep her toe in the door to come every week. What do I do? I supervise Dad. I'm on tenterhooks today because he announced to me last night that he was going to go to get his haircut at a long distance from where he lives. He's breaking the rules about why he's allowed to drive. He's supposed to drive in daylight hours in bright sunlight to the local shops. Now he's taken it upon himself to drive from Carlingford to Croydon Park. I was supposed to respond to that by saying, "I'll drive you", and I'm treading a line about freedom and all that stuff. So I'm half braced today to hear of a car accident. I wouldn't actually call that care, it's supervision, it's frustrated supervision. I'd describe it is responsibility without power and the process of doing is trying to negotiate a better sharing of power with my Mother, the care. (31)*

Some parents created stress for their carer with a constant barrage of criticism about the way the grandchildren were being reared.

> *The differences of ideas and upbringing and what I should and shouldn't do with my children, and this is where my stress level comes in. First thing when I walk in I've got my mother bombarding me with this problem and that problem and advice and do this and do that as far as my children go and that's always very difficult. That's probably more difficult than me actually doing the physical stuff. It's emotional. (30)*

The impact on the rest of the family can be considerable.

> *I think one of the other things that's important, it's very important, is the*

stress that the whole family suffers, because we are all affected. It's not only the prime carer, it's the rest of your family, my children, my husband, and, I suppose, close relatives. We haven't got them, but there's a terrible lot of stress for everybody else. (14)

The stress on a marriage or partnership is inevitable and may lead to a breakdown of that relationship. In the following case the participant was contributing to the care of the quadriplegic son of her partner. There was never any real respite, no time just with her partner and no support or understanding from the rest of the family.

That's a big thing with me at the moment, because really it's the last two months I've been really dragged under. Last Monday I came in here and just bawled my eyes out with (social worker) because I needed somebody to... because I'd had it up to here and I was ready to throw the relationship away and because it was just getting so stressful at home. (3)

Stress at work

The participants in this study were drawn predominantly from sectors of the workforce in which the work might be characterised as caring work or at least as "people oriented". Such work is typically stressful in nature. And while there are limits built into the demand placed on the paid "carer" which make a critical difference to that caring experience, it is, nevertheless, work which requires that the worker give time and attention to the needs of others, that she be available to others. This was so of the work performed by the nurses, teachers, Homecare field and office staff, human resource managers, academics and social workers who comprised the bulk of our participants. Of those who were not working in such fields, none could be said to be working in a relatively stress-free environment although one or two did "play down" the amount of stress in their own work environment and several had declined promotions or not sought such opportunities because they already had enough stress in their unpaid caring work and preferred to stay in work which had fewer responsibilities. We deal with these issues in Chapter Eight. One who had deliberately restricted her chances of advancement said...

I didn't want to take the problems from work home with me because I had enough at home to deal with. (18)

Another spoke of restricting the amount of time spent in unpaid caring work because of the nature of the paid work in which she was engaged.

> *The stresses for me are the fact that I have to work to support myself. The time I get away from work is precious and I don't know that I could handle life if I had to spend all the time when I'm not at work looking after her. That's just how I am and how our relationships are. (M)ost of my day is spent dealing directly with all the administration around aged care, frail aged people, confused people, and if I had to then in my private life to deal with that all the time as well, then I would "lose it". (29)*

A participant who worked in the personnel area emphasised the draining nature of that kind of work.

> *My job is people orientated and I suppose it would come down to too many demands on me. You just don't have the physical and emotional capabilities to deal with them all and give them sufficient time to help them adequately. And apart from that it just drains me because I don't have any time left for myself. (17)*

Relationship issues emerge again. An older generation is often unable to understand why work and career should hold such importance for women or why they might seek to improve their promotional opportunities or job choices by undertaking further study.

> *I guess in my case the main problem is my mother's total inability to acknowledge the importance of my being at work, getting to work on time and that sort of thing. She doesn't even really know or care what I do because her life is so centred on her. She makes comments about, "I suppose you are going to be far too busy this weekend" or "I know you always so busy you won't have time to come and see me". (35)*

> *Coping? Sometimes I don't cope very well at all. I feel that in terms of my father's relationship and mine, he resents me doing my university work. He doesn't like to see me as a person who's good at my career and trying to get ahead, holding other positions with the Department. He sees that as being too draining on me. What he really means is that I'm taking time away (from him). (22)*

> *I think the particular stress, especially with my parents is an expectation that they have. Because my parents lived in an era where women didn't work, they*

> *still have the attitude that a man should be able to look after his wife and they cannot comprehend that a woman would work unless she needed to financially. I use the money I earn. I love the money side. but it's not as if we're going to lose our house if I don't work. But my parents just can't take that in. (M)y sister's in the same boat. We have all the time pretended to our parents that work means nothing, takes no effort, it doesn't infringe on our family time, we're quite relaxed we don't feel tired and all that because immediately my parents would say, well you know, and take it out on our husbands, and say, "You must not work". So I guess there's that expectation that we should be available. Mind you, they're very grateful for anything we do. I'm not saying they take us for granted at all. They're very appreciative and very loving and I want to do all I can. But I guess that's the main thing. (And besides) there aren't enough hours in the day and I haven't got enough energy. (27)*

There were quite a few of our participants who spoke of the need to continue work for financial reasons and of the stress that this created especially in the current economic climate.

> *We've got an added worry at the moment in that we haven't got much work. My husband, for the first time in his life, has hardly got any work. Well, a man like he is, he's always worked hard and never had that problem and he get's very cranky and angry and I'm trying to keep him going. I haven't told my mother that he hasn't got any work because if I told her she'd be on the 'phone all the time. "Has (husband) got any work yet". And he answers the 'phone when I'm not here and she wouldn't be just doing it once in a blue moon, she'd be doing it two or three times a day. So I haven't even told her; I won't tell her. We've never had it as hard as we have now and this year has been the worst year that we've ever had. So, that's another stress. (14)*

Only one participant rejected the notion that there might be stresses associated with both working and caring.

> *I can't see any stress. No, I have never talked to anybody actually that would have stresses about it, but then I really don't ask any questions of people unless they come and tell me. (28)*

Coping with or limiting the impact of stress

Different individuals cope with the stresses in their lives in different ways and with different kinds of stress in different ways. In this study as in other research on carers, the coping strategies are various and they reveal a good deal both of the person caring and of their specific circumstances and relationships as much as they do of the particular stress of caring.

Some of the comments made in this study are about the need to be philosophical.

> *No, I'm coping and I try not to become self-pitying because that's when I really go down. But if I just take it a day at time and just think, "Well it's something that's happened and there's a lot of people in the same boat as I am". (41)*

Others set out practical steps that they had taken or strategies they had adopted.

> *In their situation it's getting worse all the time. That's the stress as far as I'm concerned. (B)asically by being very organised. That's my way of coping. (21)*

> *Make sure that you have exercise with the right food and sleep and have a balance. Like when mum was very sick, I was going swimming every single morning. And I go walking and make sure that I have a balance where I do different things and I go out to dinner and I go out to movies and I have time out for myself. (32)*

Having "time out for myself" was mentioned by others as essential. It was usually difficult to find such time. Having whole weekends away was particularly difficult but very beneficial.

> *I'm not always calm when I come home, depending on the situation when I get home. If I'm bombarded with a lot of stressful things to do with my mother, then my stress levels go up very, very high and I do feel like I'm being affected. What I've been trying to think about again is having escape weekends. I've only just started doing this lately, where I've said, "I'm going away this weekend". I left everyone, my mother and everyone, and came back very refreshed. No responsibility, no washing, no shopping, nothing like that. So, I've done that type of thing, but this is only lately. Having done it, I've felt absolutely wonderful after I've come back and thought, "Oh, I could really cope, I could really cope for the rest of the week, I could cope with anything that she says to me. Any hassles and they will just goes over my head". But if I'm really stressed my capacity to cope deserts me. (29)*

I can get very tired by the end of term, but then that's fairly much par for the course for everyone. And I have become a little more selfish, if you can use that term, at being able to just sit down and read when I feel like sitting down and reading, so I've got that time. And I garden. I'm better at doing those things that I find relaxing. The children are older, too, and they give you just that little bit more room. I'm involved in little theatre things and that's stupid really as I haven't got the time to do it, but I enjoy it and it's stimulating and so I will do that. And if I get a bit tired, well, I'd rather be tired doing that, than just being at home. No, I don't think it has effected my health. I did go through this patch last year when I thought I was depressed and then when I recognised that it was all just part of grieving. I probably was depressed but it wasn't a physiological thing. (21)

My coping strategies. How I cope on weekends, I get out of the house. I lock myself out in the backyard and the only time I come in the house on weekends is to a meal, or to sit down and have a cup of coffee and a cigarette. I don't read. I like my garden; I like my music. (3)

The importance of trying to look after yourself was a recurring theme.

You've got to stay on top yourself, otherwise you can't care for them. (12)

Friends and support within the family, particularly from a partner, made it much easier to cope. Where that support was less than unequivocal it can add to the stress.

So I feel that some of things that have helped me to cope - definitely my friends that know me. My husband has been very supportive in some ways but also very damning in others. He sees me as not being as empathetic as I could be in terms of the stress when I know that Dad's wanting me to do things for him and I feel that I don't want any more pressure in my life. (22)

Only two participants mentioned undertaking special courses specifically to assist them in coping with stress. One of these women spoke of having to "steel" herself for the decisions that lay ahead and the reaction of her father to those decisions.

I just feel that I don't cope with the guilt very well. I've done courses. I've done some insight seminars and a conflict resolution course and I've done other things where I have gone to people and colleagues to say this is the problem that I have, how can I deal with it because I am not coping very well.

> *As I said, Dad's a very strong personality. He can be very damaging and very cruel to me and I don't live with that very well and I don't know how to cope. So, emotionally I'm trying to get stronger all the time... (T)he last time he went to hospital he just really didn't want to know me, and was very nasty. And I know that when he is taken out of his home, he will see that as me pushing him and I think he's going to turn his back on me. So I think, just emotionally, I'm having to steel myself for that and I'm just trying to keep my own life together. (22)*

Several carers stated that having to be with the person they cared for all the time would be impossible. They felt that they could not cope with that.

> *If I was home with her all the time, full care, it would drive me batty, so to me work is a release from home life. Much as it's a heavy workload there too. Sometimes I go home at night and sit down and just fall asleep in front of the television because I'm so tired. (18)*

> *I couldn't do it full-time. I think I'd crack up. (3)*

Particular strategies were also mentioned. Having a "good cry" or screaming works for some or, at least, is a necessary release.

> *It's a very hard situation. I suppose I cry once a week. We have a good cry once a week and that seems to help. Sometimes I get in the kitchen and scream. I just shut the windows and scream and scream and scream, especially if I've had an argument with my mother. (14)*

Others mentioned the importance of humour.

> *A sense of humour is desperately important. We come home and we crack up. That's good. We've all got diabolic senses of humour and we all try to see the funny side. That's more difficult now because she can't really get a coherent sentence out but there are some funny things and that's important and it's important to cry. So I just think it's fairly important to be real about what's going on. Not pretend at all. That's my coping mechanism, I think. And my friends, they are great. (21)*

Those nurses we interviewed all made some mention of the fact that in their unpaid caring work they found themselves stepping into the professional role of the nurse at times. While that could help in coping with the pressure of caring for someone close to you, it also created some unease.

I think my professional role as a nurse, tells me to detach from that relationship. It's a coping mechanism, a self defence mechanism, and I find it very hard sometimes that I'm tending to do that within my family. My professional role is spilling over and that's very hard to justify, I think, for everybody including me. (19)

Religious faith was fundamental to a number in this group of carers.

I pray a lot. I'm a Christian and I accept the fact that for me God has a plan for my life and I'm available whatever crosses my path today. Well that must have been part of it. There is a beautiful verse that I hang onto that says, "They that wait upon the Lord will renew their strength. They will run and not be weary; they will walk and not faint". And I keep saying, "Hey God, don't forget the promise". However, there's also another verse in the Bible that says, "Be still and know that I am God". (Even though that was) written two thousand years ago, I see that as being very relevant, in direct relation with modern day relaxation and meditation. And so I suppose where some people when they take time to meditate and to relax might meditate on whatever, I would meditate on God, and his goodness. So, I would say I do make a conscious effort. In, I suppose, trendy language, it would be called meditation or relaxation methods. To me, it' s prayer. And it works. Well, I'm keeping going. (27)

One carer referred very frequently to the importance of meditation in her life and the difference it had brought about.

Yes, it is more stressful, but in that period of time between March last year until now I have learned an awful lot that has helped me cope with my stress levels. I'm into meditation in a big way. (If I hadn't) had the training in meditation that I had March-October, I would have been the one in need of caring rather than being the carer. That helped me with my stress, helped me to be able to cope. To be able to sit down and do meditation for fifteen to twenty minutes, sometimes ten or eleven at night, sometimes early in the morning, that's the thing that has sustained me, has made such a difference to me as a person. All the things that have happened - caring for Mum, the stress at work, the stress with my Mum - instead of it being a real peak and trough situation, it's been little peaks and little troughs.

And later...

(B)ut again I come back to my meditation and the lowering of stress and the calming of myself, understanding myself a bit better. Taking a step back and looking at the total situation from the view point of a by-stander, so to speak,

> *has made my life and health a lot better. If you can look at it from the view point of a by-stander, you can actually solve a lot of your own health and emotional problems a lot better than you can when you are caught in the situation. For me meditation is the thing that is working and I figure when you find something that is working you stick with it. I don't think I'm egotistical about it, but I'm proud of the fact that I've found something that, for me, works. (12)*

Another had also made use of meditation.

> *Yes, I'm a fairly spiritual person. I meditate. I did a relaxation course, and when I feel the need, I have a damn good cry and indulge myself there. Pick myself up and dust myself off again. There isn't anyone that I feel I can talk to. (I have) to get the strength from within myself. (37)*

The importance of inner resources was something a number commented upon.

> *My tolerance to cope with it all the time is basically that you take one day at a time. But my level of tolerance, my level of coping, I guess, (is tied to), basically her mental and physical condition at the time, whether its difficult or whether its fine. (If) she's "cool", I can cope. Basically it comes from within yourself, your level of coping. (10)*

Conclusion

Caring is stressful: it is inherently stressful work. Its stressful nature arises from the fact that one is "caring for" someone that one also "cares about", cares deeply about. That profound attention to the needs of "the other" was there even where the relationship was difficult, indeed destructive. Liking the parent had little to do with it and clearly there were times when carers did not find themselves feeling particularly loving. Stress within the relationship simply increases the stress of caring.

Caring is work. It is work from which one can never entirely "clock off". Holidays are not guaranteed and, in some cases, were rarely or never taken. There are no sick leave provisions or "flexi" days built into the caring schedule. Nor are there the protections afforded by occupational health and safety regulations. The demands are likely to increase without there necessarily being any accompanying additional support from either formal services or the rest of the family. For some carers they *are* the only family. For others, they are the only ones prepared to take on the caring role. Caring is stressful work from which one may be able to absent oneself physically for short periods but from which, emotionally, there is never an escape.

Other relationships around the carer may be problematic or may go through a "rough patch" as close relationships are inclined to do. The fact that there is a major caring demand placed on one member of the family, creates stress for others in the family as well.

For the participants in this study, caring was made more stressful by the need to juggle its demands with those of paid work. Work was important not only financially but because it represented an investment in one's own future. For many it was an escape from the demands of caring. Caring full-time was seen as an impossibility by many, if not most, of the carers in this research.

Paid work was itself stressful. The kinds of jobs in which most of our participants were engaged were, by their nature, emotionally draining: some were physically tiring as well. These jobs were "people oriented". They required the exercise of many of the same skills as in unpaid caring work. Most involved working with people who were dependent even if temporarily so, people for whose welfare the worker was held responsible. Some entailed work with elderly people who were frail, disabled or suffering from some form of dementia. Almost all were described as jobs that assumed a "giving out" or a "giving of oneself" to others, attending to the needs of others, putting one's own needs or preferences last.

So caring is stressful and paid work is stressful and family relationships and managing the home may be stressful. To take on all three is to guarantee high levels of stress even in the best of managers. At the same time, all may provide their own kinds of rewards and satisfactions. Few things are clear cut or straightforward in the fields of caring, of relationships, of love and duty, or even of working in a job you enjoy. Nevertheless, while some of our participants stated emphatically that they loved their work, no one said that they loved caring. The individual might be loved, very dearly loved, but caring holds too many emotional demands to be welcomed. And, of course, one is called upon to care when a parent or grandparent is in need of that attentive care and that will always be difficult, even distressing.

The toll on the carer's health was evident in this study as in other research. The physical toll was reflected in fatigue, headaches and in a general tendency to fall prey to whatever viruses were "going around". Back problems and hernias were also common. But the emotional toll was even greater and much more difficult to escape. Depression, anxiety, guilt, fearfulness, an inability to "shut things off", to relax, are all recorded as expressions of that emotional load.

There are important messages here for employers, service providers and policy makers. A worker carrying unreasonable loads of stress cannot work effectively. All carers will be under some stress all the time but will be having to deal with high levels of stress at particular moments when there is a crisis in relation to the health or general wellbeing of the aged relative for whom they care. The fact that they carry dual work responsibilities (and with child-care and domestic work, triple loads) means that an increase of demand in any one of these work areas, or any relationship problems, will "spill over" into the other areas of their lives and may bring them to a point of breakdown. There is not much leeway in such full, in fact overburdened, lives.

In our culture, work and private worries are to be kept separate. This is not only unreasonable, it is counter productive. It is probably accurate to say that all our participants attempted to maintain this severance, but none claimed complete success. In reality we cannot bundle up our lives in separate parcels. We cannot hope to act with equanimity in one area when things are "falling apart" in another. If we are really saying that people should be able to behave in this way, we are not simply asking for something which is not humanly possible for most people, we are seeming to approve of the kind of unfeeling, hardened, heartless automaton that might conceivably achieve it. Workers in this study who worked in environments where there was understanding of the caring loads they had to shoulder and the pain and distress that could accompany such responsibilities, were quick not only to praise their "bosses" but to say how much easier it was to carry on working and caring. They spoke of the respect for and loyalty to a manager who displayed this kind of understanding. This was so even when in reality the employer was restricted in the extent to which he or she might be able to offer more flexible working arrangements or make special provisions.

Other research has highlighted aspects of working and caring and the associated stress which we have not dwelt upon or which, as a result of the construction of the research, we are unable to examine. A number of studies, for example, have explored the different response to stress of male and female carers and concluded that women caregivers experience considerably higher levels of stress than men who work and care. Men receive more help from others than women carers and they tend to think about their responsibilities in different ways. They tend to be much more instrumental in their approach to caring, i.e., they are oriented to achieving specific goals. Also, men are "more comfortable with an authoritative teaching role" and are better able to distance themselves. One important aspect of this differing approach is their greater ability to find personal time and space away from the person for whom they care, including leaving the relative on their own. Women, on the other hand, are more inclined to conceive of caring as a reflection of their self worth. This wider research also reveals that while employed sons decreased the amount of caring they did, employed daughters did not reduce the amount of time spent with their parent and were more likely to reduce their hours of paid work or rearrange their work schedules (Neal et al. 1993).

We are not in a position to make such comparisons in this research but our findings would support the notion that women think about caring in particular ways that do seem to add to the stress that they experience. The attentiveness, the attempt to address all the needs of the parent including the parent's need to feel useful, included and as independent as was possible, shine out in these accounts. The tie with the carer's own feelings of self worth is also there. It is equally clear that it is this particular way of caring, "caring about", which added considerably to the stress load.

What we would want to add to these insights is the important recognition of the ways in which the attempt to keep separate paid work and unpaid caring responsibilities, increases the stress associated with both. It was important to our participants that they be regarded as "serious" workers for whom work and the effective performance of that work were vital parts of who they are. At the same time, it was equally important that they be able to carry out their caring responsibilities with diligence and attentiveness and that, too, was crucial to their self concept and feeling of worth.

6 Time and Caring

It is not surprising that the ways in which time is spent and the lack of time available, featured so prominently in the accounts of work and caring that our participants provided. All these women were engaged in at least two major work activities, paid work and the care of an elderly relative or relatives. Some were also still caring for children. Their days were typically very full. Time devoted to paid work is not negotiable or only marginally so and caring work had, by and large, to be fitted in around the time spent at the workplace. Not only are these two areas of work conceptualised as different, as belonging to different spheres, the worker feels compelled to kept them separate. Caring work is a private matter: how the elderly are to be cared for is something the family must resolve. In this scheme of things, neither the state nor employers nor society at large have a major responsibility for unpaid caring work in the private domain. Unpaid caring activity and its emotional demands are to be kept separate from, should not impinge upon, the world of work. As detailed in the previous chapter, the very effort to keep separate two demanding, indeed preoccupying, areas of their lives, created considerable stress for the majority of the carers in this study.

Caring is time consuming. For workers, therefore, time must be found wherever they can, and that, of course, means making effective use of every bit of time that is not already consumed by work. Other implications flow from this. A worker who has a major responsibility of care must be well organised. She must also, almost inevitably, devote time to caring that would in different circumstances be given over to self, to hobbies, to further study, to recreation. It may mean that caring for a parent takes up time that would otherwise be spent with other family members - children, a partner.

The issue of recreation time and leisure in the lives of carers must await another book but it should be acknowledged at this point how important, for most workers, is that non-work time. This parcel of time is seen as time to recover, to escape from the pressures of work. It is viewed as the reward for work. It is considered a right and a necessity. How else could one keep working but with regular time off?

Most of the women in this study had little time which was their own and what time there was, was often gained at some cost as will be seen in the following accounts. The need to be well organised, to manage one's time as effectively as possible also involved a cost and created additional strains. There is little possibility of being idle just for once or of doing something frivolous or spontaneous. The accounts point yet again to the wide range of tasks and responsibilities that caring roles entail, to tight schedules and the set routines that need to be followed.

> *We've gone through stages where I've done all the housework, mowed the lawns, done the gardening, looked after her, done all the washing, ironing, all at once. I'd try and do all those things and still spend quality time with her and if I was doing all these things she would say, "We're not spending time together". With working, sometimes I don't get home until six o'clock and you really want to crash and you feel like saying how about we have "Kentucky Fried". If you looked in my fridge you would find very little food. Basically, all our food goes straight into her fridge because we eat together in the evening and it's easier to have the whole lot in one place and go over and prepare it there rather than taking it across. We can actually be talking while I'm preparing it, if I'm preparing it in there with her.(12)*

> *I don't hang around, wandering around the shops or go and visit a friend during my time off. I feel like there's a real need to come home immediately and I didn't realise how strong that was until we had three days when Mum had gone into Respite before we went away on holidays and I spent all day still going to the window peering up to the back garden. We'd get up during the night to go to the loo or something and we'd be (going) to the back door (to check on mother), both of us... I would never think to go off after school with the others down to the pub for a drink on a Friday because, a) I've got children to come home to any way, but b) there's that sense that I've got to come home and check that there's no disaster. (21)*

> *Sometimes at seven o'clock at night when I've done the shopping and piling it into the basket, I think, "Why am I doing this? I don't want to be doing this at this hour of the night". But that's okay. Tomorrow morning it's done and you don't have to do it again for another few weeks. (33)*

> *Go home, eat, get showered, go to bed and get up in the morning, back to work. Weekends - my parents and my daughters, and that's it. (24)*

> *I'm doing my degree now and I've taken two subjects, so, there is a lot of study time. I have to wake up at four o'clock in the morning (and work) until six thirty to do my study. This is* ***my*** *time. Then I have to get ready, prepare things for the night time. The kids go to school. And then (at the end of the day), you get home and you've got to either cook dinner and you've got their*

> *emotional things that happened during the day, some drama, and then you've got your mother to ring up at eight thirty. So at night time you really can't do any study. And then you've got the weekend which is taken by shopping, housework. Sunday afternoon when I might otherwise have a bit of free time to spend with my kids, or friends, I can't have that because that's the time that I have allocated for my mother, every week and my family life is suffering because I can't spend much time with my kids. My kids are really suffering because I'm a sole parent and they need that back up. I can (only) give them that between say six to eight of a night time and that's hard with teenagers because they are not around (for long). (41)*

These are full lives indeed! But the busyness is almost all "other-directed", a response to the needs of others. It is difficult and costly to have time to one's self. To pursue one's own goals may mean even tighter schedules or less sleep.

And here, too, is that recurring theme of caring as a constant preoccupation, an ever present anxiety about the parent or grandparent. This is an important part of what is entailed in "caring about" someone. The other part is the attempt to ensure there is "quality time" spent with the person, listening, paying attention to them. As other writers have pointed out this means that the carer "must be present or readily available". It requires that they not be "too preoccupied with their own activities". It "fragments time": it "imposes a severe restriction on the carer's thoughts, let alone their activities" (Land 1991, p.12). When you carry a major responsibility of care, you very often lack the power of choice not to be so involved in the time consuming and draining activities described here. And the activities such as study, something for one's self but most especially an investment in one's future, are particularly problematic. How is one to concentrate on writing an essay let alone a thesis, in such circumstances?

> *Fragmentation of time, the fact that I'm never guaranteed of carrying through and completing anything I start in any type of career... Because I'm a very experienced teacher, I'm managing the teaching here on my ear. No problems, easy! The research is another story altogether. The task of writing a book when three people are dividing the labour and coming together for a day, talking, sparking off each other, no problem, except that it took longer than it should have. The thesis is another matter altogether. I'm too fragmented. I start something, I start on a train of thought, and a crisis occurs, and I have to go and live there, carting (all my) stuff around (with me). My concentration is fragmented. (31)*

> *Sometimes it just overwhelms you. You can feel yourself start to slip backwards. You say, "Oh, another bill to pay when am I going to find the time to do this". I've got a bad habit of putting it in my handbag ready to pay and I forget about it, all because I am so busy doing other things. I'm far too preoccupied. I'm thinking of too many things. I even find when I'm talking to people I'm saying two words together because I'm trying to get it all out in a rush. So there is too much going on and I don't have time to concentrate to get it all done properly to my satisfaction and they're all demanding things, all demanding. They all have to be done. Most of them have an emotional impact and whether it's there and then or whether it's afterwards that it actually hits you... But, yes, they've all got (an) emotional (toll), and I'm finding the emotions are really dragging. (17)*

To discuss how time is spent with a group of carers is to begin to understand the stress, the tensions, that permeate their lives. There is never enough time.

> *I just wish I had more hours in the weekend. I really would wish they'd extend the weekend. (3)*

> *My worst enemy is time. If I had some financial back up then I would be able to say, "Well, I can only work four days a week and I want to have one day with my mother". But I haven't got that and that's where I haven't got the time. Time is money. (41)*

> *Not enough time and I guess the most difficult thing is keeping everyone happy and making everyone in that circle of your interest feel that they are the most important and the most cared for without forgetting to care for yourself a little bit. (27)*

Because time is short, the need to establish priorities, and ration time spent on some activities, becomes an essential strategy. We asked our participants how they managed their time, how they fitted in the myriad of tasks, how they negotiated any competing demands. Some researchers have objected to the use of the term "juggling time" (Howe 1993) but our participants when asked whether or not it was an apt description of the experience of caring, were, almost without exception, very ready to apply the phrase to their own situation. For most, such notions as "over lapping roles" (Vanden Heuvel 1993), for example, seemed a rather inadequate way to conceptualise what they experienced day-by-day.

"Juggling" is the right word. I sort of have this mental picture of about five different things up in the air. Your family, your friends, your job, the person you are caring for, your social life,... you've got all these things up in the air and you can only hold one at a time, not two, one. You throw them all up and you hope which one is going to come down next. Like this circumstance this evening. I'm juggling Mum up in the air somewhere and I'm here talking to you, you're the thing I've got in my hand at the moment, and I should have spent another couple of hours at work before I came home, so that's up in the air and I should have done some more washing this evening, so that's up in the air, all these things. So it is literally a juggling act... It's tiring and it's one of those things that you look at and think, one of these days I'm going to miss and all those balls that are up in the air are going to fall on top of my head and all I'm going to be able to do is go "help" and cover my head. (28)

As a result certain things have to go; one can only "juggle" so much at any one time. Some things are just let slip, but in other cases the decision to drop particular activities or aspects of one's life is very consciously made.

I know I'm eating (more), I know I'm sleeping more, because actually when you said who misses out, the kids have missed out on my time, but my time with them has been more quality time. So I sort of put myself to bed early so I get a good seven hours sleep so I'm not yelling and screaming at them. I'm not coping; I am under stress. Very early on in the piece, I made a concerted effort that something had to go. Professionally it was my Masters and socially it was friends, and people think that's crazy, but something has to go. You say how do you cope, actually that's how I coped. We just don't - of course we have gone to the odd dinner party, but we haven't entertained, it's just out of the question. (36)

The struggle to cope with the competing demands, to allocate time and attention to all those requiring it, created considerable stress for most of the participants in this study.

I always try to be in two places at once. Which is pretty hard, but you try to cover up one, let your Mum know that everything's fine and let your husband know that she needs you desperately and you have to be there. Pretty tricky. For example, if I go with my Mum to a doctor and you know the appointment is at two o'clock and you know your husband gets home at four o'clock and the doctors are running late, and you keep looking at the watch... You know when he gets home, he's not going to kill you, but you're not there. "Oh, she's not here because she's with her Mum"!! So you sort of get all worked up inside because you have to be there with your Mum but you have to be home

> *when your husband comes. You can't be, just like at the same time. (23)*

> *Negotiating people's different needs. I'm finding (that) the emotional, responsibility, the practical responsibility, the fatigue, the time demands... Really when you list them, you think why would you do it? Both my mother and mother-in-law are really quite demanding. The emotional demand is terrible, really terrible. (16)*

And the ever present anxiety that is part and parcel of "caring about" can, at times, be acute and make it impossible to concentrate on one's job.

> *I would say that one of the things that gets me is the anxiety of having the hostel ring and say your Mum's not well, and then you have to try and cope with your work and still keep on with what you are doing here, (while) your mind is somewhere else and you are waiting to get there. (8)*

The intrusion into work time of one's caring responsibilities and the feeling of being distracted by caring worries while at work, created additional stress and guilt. Workers who are carers feel torn between the two roles and the time and energy they can or should devote to each.

> *Feeling guilty that you have to make excuses all the time to leave. I've got to get home because this is going on. (19)*

> *It's hard to cope with. Sometimes you just have to say to yourself, "Well, I'm human, two arms, two legs. I'm doing the best I can do". Yet you are constantly questioning yourself, am I doing the right thing with my work? Am I really doing the right thing? Am I being selfish? Should I really be at home doing what I was doing for the past few years? It's very easy to get into that negative state, very easy, very easy, and that's one thing that I keep juggling. I keep asking myself, "Am I doing the right thing?" (15)*

Some expressed their dilemma as one of attempting to fit caring around their work; others of trying to fit their paid work around their caring. In all these accounts, the stated need to keep separate the two major spheres of their lives is tellingly expressed.

> *I try and keep it separate. I like to think that I come in here and do my work and do it well and keep the hostel side of it separate. I do a lot of things for my Mum on the weekends.(8)*

Up until now it hasn't been too bad. Now she's hospitalised, I'm going in the morning before work and after work and if I need to juggle the times a bit I can because of flexi-time. It hasn't really been a big problem. But in the future, if her health deteriorates and she needs more help, I haven't thought in terms of me not working and helping her more. I've only thought in terms of me being able to buy the services I need for her because I can't not work... So I'd have to work more to buy the services to supplement what I can't do because I'm working. It's that vicious cycle. (29)

With medical appointments you do need to just find extra time and I find working in an organisation like this, because we have flexi-time, it is easier to think about it. But it's still a bit of a conflict sometimes. I have used annual leave when I was looking for the nursing home. (1)

I have to make sure I don't get too involved with afternoon groups on the afternoons that I know that I'm going to go and see Mum because they (in the hostel) go to dinner at five o'clock. Now if I leave here at four thirty, there's only a half an hour and then she doesn't want me to go and that sort of thing. I'm better off looking at trying to get away early some days, and things like taking your flexi-day to take her for new glasses and things like that. I don't know what I'd do if I couldn't get flexi-days, when I have to do things like that. (8)

Well, the home demands are the most difficult really, because I need my job, so I have to put the workplace first and cope with the other later. (18)

A number of the carers in this group had specifically chosen to work part-time so as to have greater flexibility, more time for caring and less stress.

It's quite a heavy (teaching) load. Basically, last year, I would have had a whole afternoon off and virtually a whole morning off and the rest of the time, the days were so broken up - I mean I can do things in them, I can go and pay bills... Yes, it's the flexibility. So I get those things done during the day. Any time off I have is my own time, so that's good and I enjoy that. Well I couldn't manage without it. I couldn't do it full-time, there's no way. I couldn't do it full-time primarily because of the responsibilities of caring for Mother. (21)

Several spoke of using leave provisions. One spoke of holding on to her long service leave in anticipation of the need to use it in the future to look after her mother in a more intensive way.

Long term I feel that I'm hanging on to my long service in case... And I feel personally whatever is going to happen, would probably happen within an eight to nine month period anyway. If there was a more sudden deterioration than we've already been through and I feel it would reach the stage where she would realise that now was the time. We are very lucky in the sense that I'm still single. Had I just been married, not even had kids, I would not have been able to give her as much time as I do. (12)

Another had considered cutting down on working hours but in the end had decided to place both parents in a nursing home. It was not an easy decision to make.

I thought at one stage I probably would have to cut it down, or give up working, when I had both of them at home to cope with. That time was very, very hard for me. So they suggested I put them in a home: "It would be easier for you". At first it was very hard to do it. But I did it. (24)

The lack of time to one's self in a recurring theme in this research as in other research on carers. One's own needs are very often the last to be considered and it is a difficult lesson to learn that unless one does attend to one's own needs then there is a real chance that one will "burn out" and cease to be of use to anyone.

Time for self. The biggest stress is lack of time. Lack of time to do what I have to do to earn a buck. (4)

You're putting yourself last, that's a typical woman I think. Well I don't know if it's typical woman, but you find that because you've got responsibilities you've got to put other people first and somewhere along the line you put yourself last. (30)

Trying to be more organised, doesn't seem to work. What I find now, I try not to listen too much to everybody else's needs. I've come to the decision that I've got needs too and that really to make everybody else happy, I have to have some of mine made happy as well. I basically had to say to the family, "Okay, you've had your turn, now it's mine", and put my foot down in some cases and say, "You lot are a bit greedy. How about me?" (40)

In some of the accounts there was a good deal of "give and take". That not only makes caring easier, it also means that it is more likely the carer will be able to find some time for herself. In other situations the carer was constantly giving and her time was never her own.

There is one final comment on the importance of time in this study. How time is perceived is dependent on the whole context in which one is living out one's life. Carer's lives are typically very full and stressful. For those who work full-time or near to full-time in the paid workforce as well as carrying a major responsibility of care for an aged relative, the pressure can be very great. That pressure is experienced as the attempt to fit as much as possible into a fixed number of hours. Time is thus a precious commodity. The aged, on the other hand, tend to experience time in a very different way and to have little perception as to the tight schedules within which their carer is "operating".

> *And the slowness of it too. It's very hard when you are going at a hundred miles an hour all week, to suddenly, I mean that's hard for them to cope with too, that you are going a hundred miles an hour. For example, when we went to... a funeral in Canberra on Friday and came back on Monday, it took me six hours to get from Canberra to Camden because Mother had her camera and she wanted to take pictures of the blossom trees and the wattle trees... And my daughter said, "So what, Mum, that's all right. Gran doesn't go out often. Just let her do it". And I thought, the kids are often better than I am at slowing down. It's the slowing down that makes it hard. (35)*

Among many women of an older generation there is little understanding of what participation in the workforce entails and, most especially, what it means for a woman who will also be carrying the domestic load and child care as well as attending to the needs of the parent. Time is not the same thing for people in very different circumstances.

Time as a moral issue

To discuss time is to discuss what we value and so is a vital issue in any consideration of caring for the elderly and most particularly in the context of work and caring. The "valuing" of some activities (and therefore of time spent in them) over other tasks and goals is the context in which caring is carried out. How we use our time is often cast in moral terms. Time is precious; we should use it profitably. It is seen to be a measure of the kind of person we are, not just in the obvious sense that we have a particular "occupation" but again in moral terms, in terms of our value as human beings. Yet as a community, while we pay lip service to the importance and morality of caring, we place less value on caring work in the paid workforce than we do on those jobs tied to money, to making decisions about financial matters and directing the economy or generating wealth. As for unpaid caring work, necessary though it be, we have given it almost no recognition at all. Caring for others is supposed to be a worthy occupation but there is little public recognition and no monetary reward. It is to be undertaken for love not money and therefore, paradoxically, it is both a most esteemed *and* greatly undervalued activity.

Time is money. That means that time spent in simply being there for someone, being available, listening time, companionable time, is less and less likely to be recognised as important by service providers. This is so in spite of a recognition that it is this kind of time that is highly valued by the elderly, especially those still living in their own homes or in nursing homes. If companionable time is to be provided as a service, then it must be a volunteer service. Where a cost is involved, there must be something that can be shown for the time spent with a client.

What have we to show for time spent in caring for elderly parents? Where are those prized "tangible outcomes"? There is very little to show that can be seen and "valued" by others. The care of children may produce adults of whom we can feel proud. What of the care of the elderly? And, at a personal level, if our time has been fragmented by the very business of caring, then it is unlikely we will have much to show that will bring reward in the form of promotion or increased income or a more prestigious job.

Those who do not spend time in caring work and especially those who are not expected to care, are, in general, the "gainers" in our society at least in terms of money, status, power, independence, control over their lives, having more choices and, as a result, having a more secure future.

This is in no way to denigrate caring for the elderly. On the contrary, it is to underline what we all recognise as the hypocrisy that attaches to the way we value certain kinds of occupations over others and the rewards that we confer on these activities and jobs as a result. In immediate terms, carers are the losers: but we all lose (eventually) in this way of the world. This is so not just because we will all get old and may need to be cared for, for short or longer periods, but because of the skewing or distorting of all our values in a way that is ultimately destructive of community and human good.

Conclusion

The carers in this study are shouldering a major responsibility of care in an era in which the values outlined above are seemingly in the ascendancy in all areas of life. It is also a period when paid work and especially secure, long term work, is in short supply. Thus to have to give up work or take up a more vulnerable position in the workforce because of increasing caring responsibilities, holds even greater dangers than in the past. While older women seem to have fared better in finding new employment than have older male workers who lose their jobs (for whatever reason), the current employment situation remains a risky one for all workers over forty five (Freeland 1997).

Along with high rates of unemployment has developed another and contrary trend. Those in paid employment are working longer and longer hours. These extended hours at work are represented as productivity gains (Probert 1993). For carers the pressure to work longer hours and do more in their paid work comes at a time when they find themselves needing more time and energy for that other job - the care of an elderly relative. If they are to do both jobs and remain in the workforce (their investment in their own future), they will need greater support from community services. But the community sector is being cut back in ways that mean that workers who are carers are to receive fewer and fewer services. If they want support from formal services, they will have to pay. It is our view that most of the workers in this study would not be in a position to pay for the services they will need if they are to continue both to work *and* to care.

It is to state the obvious but perhaps we need to do that in this kind of study... time spent in caring cannot be valued in the same way as time spent in many other jobs. The value of caring cannot be measured in money terms although, as we point out in our concluding chapter, it saves the community vast sums of money every day of the year.

Caring time operates within a different framework from that of the paid workforce. One does not clock on and off. There are no flexi-days or sick leave or other accrued leave. Usually, you are not in a position to hand over to someone else when your part of the task is completed. There is no one else to take overall responsibility, or to "take the rap".

Caring time does not have the same kinds of tangible outcomes as time spent in other kinds of work although a number of our carers spoke of the personal satisfaction they felt in seeing their parent or parent-in-law well looked after or with a renewed self confidence.

Caring time is fractured and fragmented time. Much of caring is just being there or being available when needed. It always involves an emotional component even in the performing of simple physical tasks and even when not in the presence of the one who is being cared for. Time spent in caring can thus be more stressful and physically and emotionally more draining than much paid work.

7 Reflections on Caring

The women in this study were included because they were carrying a major responsibility of care for an elderly relative while at the same time working full-time (or near to full-time) in the paid workforce. As will become clear in succeeding chapters, work was of importance to the women in this study. It was important for financial reasons, because it represented an investment in their own future and thus a degree of security for the remainder of their lives, and because they enjoyed their work and considered it an important part of their identity. But their unpaid caring work was also of great importance. It had not been taken on lightly and it also constituted a significant part of their identity even when, as a few specified, they had never considered themselves as being "by nature" a carer.

As we have already noted, it was the caring responsibilities that featured in these accounts. Paid work appeared to be, by and large, the least complicated part of their lives. On the one hand, its emotional demands were more manageable. On the other hand, any physical demands were often directly tied to the difficulties of trying to accomplish the great range of tasks that they found themselves having to perform in all the other areas of their crowded lives. So it is not surprising that they reflected in more detail upon their caring responsibilities and on what they had learnt as a result of the experience of shouldering a major caring load. In addition, we had explicitly asked them what advice they might give to someone who was considering taking on a major responsibility of care. In this chapter we examine both those general ideas about caring and the suggestions that were made as to how it might be managed.

Ideas about caring

Many of these reflections were of a general and philosophical nature. Some of our participants spoke of their own strongly held religious beliefs and the essential link between these and the choices they had made in relation to taking on responsibility for the care of an elderly relative.

> *I just know that I'm happy that I've got Mum. I'd hate to lose her even though she's stopping me doing what I want. The thought of her going, I can't accept*

at the moment. Maybe my cousin is right, because I'm a religious person and I value things on the human side, like caring and loving each other, maybe that is how I am made. But there's a lot of work to do out there in the community. And those people who are bored at home, I'd have an advice for them. Get out of your own surroundings and go out there and you can do so much good for the community. (11)

The notion that charity begins at home was also evoked.

My daughter went to a nursing home to work and used to come home so depressed because she said, "It's incredible, they are forgotten, they are just lying there waiting to die and they've got family but they are never there, or only for two minutes". She met a lady that really made a profound impact on her because this lady, there was not a thing wrong with her, only a slight stroke, and she was in this horrible home with Alzheimers and incontinent people around her and her daughter lives in this street in a mansion. Only her and her husband and the house is empty. How can you justify that? How can I justify putting my Mother away with three bedrooms upstairs? How can I justify myself before God, before myself, or my children? Can you understand my point of view? I couldn't live with myself. Charity begins at home, don't you agree? (11)

One women spoke about the obligation to care as a moral obligation.

I have a moral obligation to my parents because, after all, they gave me life in the first place. It is a matter of balancing their quality of life against my right to work. (39)

To others in the group the issue of responsibility and where it lies was not seen in quite such straightforward ways. Some spoke of guilt and the way that families play upon guilt. They felt very strongly that families (which so often means particular women) should not be made to feel that they must take on the role of carer.

Things like the loss of privacy, the recognition of the strain it puts on the individual relationships within families. The rose coloured cottage kind of pie-in-the-sky, crap you hear. Everyone loves each other and the family is a wonderful institution. A lot of that needs a few realistic holes dropped through it. And I suppose the other thing is, again, people shouldn't be made to feel that they have to take on the caring role. If you chose to do it , fine but if you chose to do it but then find you can no longer continue to do it, then there ought to be some way of ensuring help for you and genuine alternatives... without feeling like you've failed. (9)

The emphasis on the importance of family care is clearly there in all the accounts but equally there is a call for far greater recognition of the strains that it places upon both the carer and her family and of the need for viable and acceptable alternatives to co-resident caring.

I think this has been, in one way, good for our children that they will have had some memory of that. We don't care, in our society, basically we are so dislocated from our families. I think there must be a lot of people around who have a terrible sense of guilt that their parents live there and they live here and they've had to go into a home. In a sense I will look back on this time, I think, thankful that I've been able to take that care of my mother. She did it for me as a child. I see it as part of a whole cycle of life, but it isn't something that you expect. Everybody's situation is probably different. (21)

I feel as if I've resolved a lot of my resentments. I love my mother very much. I worry as much about their quality of life as my own. I think my mother's quality of life is "ratshit". I feel that she should have more companionship and she shouldn't be left to rattle around in the house by herself. Her dementing is partly caused by the lack of inter-personal contact. I don't necessarily think I'm a person that can supply that. I used to feel really guilty. (31)

The need for greater recognition of what caring entails was a recurring theme - recognition from the rest of the family, from professionals, from employers and from the community at large. Providing quality of life for the elderly, ensuring as great a degree of independence as possible for as long as possible, is very often based upon the expectation that caring responsibilities will be picked up by families and particularly by the women in those families. The emotional load is rarely acknowledged.

Yes, I think recognising it as a real issue. The health services have put a lot of money into (helping) people stay out of nursing homes and (remain) in their (own) home, which ideologically is a wonderful idea, but it's people like me who have to help out in those situations. And it's the emotional drain. I really don't think that the washing and the ironing and the cooking and all that are a big deal. Lets face it, today they take an hour to put on. (36)

Well I just think it is that the population is ageing. The pressure to look after the aged in their homes theoretically is fine but practically is very hard. It's very hard. Employers need to be aware that this is a real issue. And I really have to say, I think, maybe I've just been affected because of the time, it's happening to me now, I think it is a far more important issue than maternity leave. (36)

Caring and self knowledge

Caring responsibilities for an elderly parent tend to come upon one in the latter part of one's own life. There is an increasing recognition that there are in fact many elderly carers looking after still more elderly parents. But this study has focused on workers who are carers. For such carers, what is of overriding importance is where they are in their own careers, and the extent to which their jobs are secure. A number commented on the fact that they were at a stage in their own careers when fitting in extra responsibilities for frail parents was more readily managed than would have been the case at as earlier point in their working lives.

(I)n many ways I've got off extremely lightly in that my father has lasted to over ninety and my mother may well hit ninety herself. So, that this has come to me at a time when my career is established and I'm perhaps more confident and secure in what I'm prepared to do. My sister has had a much worse time of it. To a certain extent because she's in a woman's job, as a person she's not perhaps seen as a real worker by her husband or her parents or her demanding children, or perhaps by herself. She's had a lot more pressure on her and a lot less say in how things go. (39)

For others the caring load was particularly difficult to fit into their lives. They had continuing responsibility for care of children and many had demanding and stressful jobs. The lack of preparedness for what elder care might involve was noted, as indeed the lack of any real acknowledgment that ageing will involve some adjustments for both the aged and those that care about them. As a society we have not shown ourselves particular adept at dealing with ageing in realistic and honest ways.

As I wrote my letter to friends at Christmas, I made some comment about how it's probably a good thing you don't know, early in life, what lies ahead of you and yet I wonder if there should be some preparation. Maybe when you are young you can't hear it anyway. You don't believe your parents are ever going to get old, but it comes as quite a shock, I think, when it happens. I've suddenly got a whole group of friends where similar things are happening to them and we aren't prepared for it in any way. We're not prepared and we have got an ageing population. Whether there needs in some sense to be an awareness raising to people in their thirties that this is going to happen. I don't know. It just is something that I suppose you just put it out there and think, "I'll deal with it when I come to it". But you never quite think it's going to be there. But then maybe that's true of all these things in life. We're not prepared for parenthood, nobody prepares us for that. (21)

Quite a number of our participants were working in caring jobs, some in aged care. They commented on the particular difficulties in caring for one's own parent and how that is not always appreciated by those outside the situation.

I think they take it for granted because I'm a carer and I think, probably, my friends take it that I will cope with this because it's my job, as well. I mean I'm looking after everyone else's parents, well why can't you look after your own. I remember when I had my first child and I had worked in nurseries at hospitals before and thought, well, I've looked after twenty four babies, it will be a snack. I'll have no problems. And yet I was the first one to be howling my eyes out day and night because I couldn't cope. And I think it relates the same. It's much more difficult to (deal with your own parent). I mean I can organise anyone else's parents and get all the care, support and all of that, but I can't with my own. (27)

Another commented on how important that training in nursing had been in enabling her to cope even though it could never entirely prevent her responding as a daughter at particular moments and feeling the distress very acutely because of that close relationship.

My brothers admit that their wives can't cope. They can stand Mum for a week to two weeks and that's the limit. And as it is they live both ends of the country so Mother couldn't physically travel to be with them anyway. But when they did take her for short breaks their level of tolerance is a lot lower than mine and they are very grateful to send her back home. They're very good with her but they smother her because they fear, they don't understand. So she's got greater freedom with me. But then, on the other hand, she manipulates them more than she can manipulate me. So the ideal situation is a nurse in every family to have the responsibility because the patient is dealt with more fairly, has a better level of life... I can be quite objective. But education of the disease helped me to be objective. I had to divorce the subservient daughter of that generation to the authoritative nurse here. Definitely, I had to find myself and then admit that I had downfalls. There was one night when Mum collapsed that there was also me, the person, and not necessarily the nurse. (10)

One women spoke of the far greater understanding she now had for those caring for their own parents and of the fraught nature of that relationship. She also dwelt on the impersonal nature of much institutional care and the accompanying loss of identity. This needs to be understood by all who work in such environments.

I have much greater understanding of the dilemmas for caring sons and daughters of the very ambivalent feelings that that creates for them towards their elderly parents. That sort of feeling of honour but also a feeling of dislike because of the different people they are and the very demanding people they are. So I think that it enables me at least to understand those other staff. Sometimes I think, "God, what's wrong with so-and-so that they're not interested in caring for this old person, how awful"... You realise what a really ambivalent situation it is for most people. It also helps me to understand the conflict that arises between sons and daughters with regard to the care of their parent. I mean I can't really rely on my brother for help with my Mother but sometimes I wish I could. And I often see families with three or four middle-aged children who bicker with one another and fight about who is providing more care or who isn't and who won't do their bit and I think it just heightens my awareness of all of that. It also heightens my awareness of the terrible difficulties for elderly people living longer and having to live in situations which really for them are very (distressing). They are losing their identity. My mother, I think, feels as though she's totally lost her identity living in that situation because there's nobody that knows any of her past. So she can't sit down and talk about old times, old friends. I mean nobody knows who they are... It also heightens my awareness of how centred elderly people become, how small their world becomes as a phenomenon and how difficult that is also for carers to deal with, just cope with that. I think there are very few elderly people that don't go into that narrowing phase which becomes very self-centred again. So yes I think it's certainly made a difference in terms of the skills (that I have acquired). (35)

The gains that flowed from the experience were also detailed.

You get a lot of satisfaction out of caring, depending on the type of person you are. I do, that's why I went into nursing. You do get a lot of satisfaction out of caring for someone, not just - it is emotional - but I think you are fulfilling, maybe it's a mothering instinct, I don't know. I just think the best thing is just do it and get on with it and things will get better. If it's a really hard time, (it is important to remember that) sometimes it is not, sometimes it can be a very pleasant... (40)

And there is much to be gained from the elderly themselves.

So there are quite a few things to be learned, quite a few things. (S)he's (grandmother) very strong. I see myself in that, and it feels good. Her expressions, her moods, her humour. My goodness! And she's such a hopeless romantic. She's like the Bill Collins of Greece. She'll watch these Greek videos and then - she can't see them very well - she'll put the voices up, and she's away. It's true, it's true. Something that amazes me about my grandmother is her never-ending youthfulness in a way. Some days she's two hundred and fifty years of age and then when she puts these films on she's like a child or a teenager. It's good, it's good. (15)

Self knowledge and maturity are referred to, an ability to be more gentle both with one's self and with others. It is also important to know when you need a break and to recognise the signs of excessive stress.

I recognise now, when I'm involved with the P&C (Parents and Citizens Association), and it's a fairly large school so you are dealing with a lot of parents and you are dealing with a lot of teachers, that I'm not as offended by people's responses as maybe I might (once) have been. Maybe, again, it's just maturity, but I recognise that often people's angry or uncomfortable responses in a meeting situation are not necessarily directed at me or at someone else. I think, too, there has certainly been a greater acceptance of myself, just the frailty. I think when you are a competent person it can be fairly scary for a while to find that you appear to be very frail and fragile in certain areas, and I guess that's part of the grieving process too. I went to a grief counselling course last year and I recall one thing they said. "One of the symptoms was that you are intensely sad." And I thought, "Ah, I'm not mad, depressed, I'm just sad". To be in that place and to know that's (how it is) and that lots of people around me are living like that all the time. It just makes you gentler on other people. (21)

Knowledge of self. You get to know where you are strong, where you are not strong and you become aware of when you need time out. Managing all the jobs because there are quite a lot of physical jobs involved and emotional work as well. Becoming aware of your feelings is quite important. Getting stronger. People who had no idea, they'd sort of seen themselves in that very female role, the passive, submissive whatever, over the years, never worked in a workforce, are quite amazed, some of them, about how they are coping.

> *They actually manage to pull it off, this massive work load, this massive emotional strain and they are doing it and surviving. It's not a one way street either. They get stuff back from the loved one, they get appreciation, sometimes they don't, sometimes their loved one is a pain in the neck. Then they come and talk about it at the carers' group. (4)*

> *I think having said to you that I don't acknowledge stress, I acknowledge stretch. I'm stretched!! If what you want to do, you want to do well, you have to have a mental attitude towards it and it can't be encumbered by a lot of other things that you are calling stressors, because you won't do what you want to do properly. So when I talk about balance, it's maintaining what you set out to be your plans. The people you are caring for are a part of your life, (but) the most important part of life is your immediate family, your husband and your job. They all have a place and sometimes, maybe, it just works. I think it would probably be a lot harder if your children were young and you were attempting to do what I'm doing. But I think the same principle applies. I mean I've got workers who are studying and they've got children too and providing they take all those things into account and how it is for them, they shouldn't burn out. But you've got to be aware that you can because as they say, I don't think modern woman says what is enough. We just keep doing a little bit more and a little bit more. (33)*

Other kinds of understanding were also mentioned.

> *(T)hat you don't take your age for granted, because every year that passes, it's never coming back. A lot of people my age don't have that gift... Sometimes I'm twenty two and sometimes one hundred and fifty and that's because I've been with an old person so long. (A)ppreciating what you've got because our bodies for example, how we treat ourselves, they will start talking to us later, sooner or later. We're not like a vehicle that's got spare parts. What you see is what you get. Age. Sometimes I envy the old person their wisdom and how wise they are and how much they know and I'd give anything just to (have that now). Actually sometimes she (grandmother) says to me, so, how old are you really? It's like a reverse role play. (15)*

Others also mentioned the need to keep a balance, to keep things in proportion.

> *I think keeping everything relative and accepting that this is the day that I've got and (focus on) what I (need to) get done today. I'm not going to be worried about what I failed at yesterday and I'm not going to worry about what I might have to face tomorrow. And I think that has been a great*

learning experience through having teenagers actually... And in seeing life in day-by-day, sometimes minute-by-minute (terms), I think that's something that I've learned to do and so I guess there's a lot less anxiety there than probably ten years ago. (27)

I suppose each day is a bonus, while I can do what I want to do, and while they are still okay. (33)

The fact that what you are having to negotiate in the caring role is a new relationship was something else that merited comment. All the relationships in which you are involved will need to be re-negotiated.

If my long standing friend hadn't been so self-effacing; had (he) made any demands on me, I don't know what I would have done. (I'd have) had to drop him. I should say that I get a lot of love and support from my parents. From my father I get some understanding of my situation. He's not dealing with it realistically because of his need to maintain his own self-esteem, and deny his ageing, but he is conscious of my situation and he wants to help me. And from my mother I just get heaps and heaps of love, affection, gratitude and some knowledge through the dementia of my needs. So it's very positive too, it's a new relationship. (31)

This carer also spoke of the considerable problems that were involved in attempting to ensure quality of life for both her parents and most particularly her mother who was suffering from fairly advanced dementia. It was difficult for a daughter to negotiate those new relationships and thus provide the needed support. But relying upon formal services to step in was, in her view, completely unrealistic. Community services were not in a position to provide adequate back-up.

There have been times when I've had terrible conflicts with him (father) in an attempt to crash through and I've found it counter productive because there's too much "shit" around from the daughter in the parent - daughter relationship. So I don't actually think it should come back onto the daughters to be the ones. The parent has too much to lose too. The community service people say to me, "You've got to back off so that we can come in". But I think that's really simplistic because the attempts that I have made to "back off", sometimes I've cracked and I've gone to see surreptitiously how they are getting on and I've walked in on situations of chaos. To me they seem like chaos, no food in the house, two old people at dinner time curled up in a foetal position sleeping in different parts of the house in obvious exhaustion

> *at bickering at each other and chaos. And serious car accidents, there have been two of them. Maybe I should just be tougher and let it go, but I don't want that responsibility. It's not going to be picked up (by community services). My mother is the defenceless one in all this. What the community care people say is that my situation, my parent's situation, they live in a palace; they are really well looked after; my father's coping really well compared with most old people. Well, I think, if that's the case, the quality of life of old people is absolutely "ratshit" and I don't want to see that happen to my parents. I don't want to see that happen to my little mother. Somebody has to bite the bullet but I don't know how. (31)*

Who is in the best position to offer good care and who are the best carers, were also issues that were explored. A few of the women reflected on their own capacities to care and what being "caring" might mean.

> *I think I'm a very organised person. I don't think that I could do what I do unless I was organised. I have always been a competent sort of person. I don't tackle things if I don't believe I can be competent at it. So I don't play sport, for example. I find a challenge in the whole caring thing in that I believe I care competently and it's probably the emotional area where I feel like I'm not as loving as I would desire to be. I don't believe that I'm actively not loving but I recognise in my heart there are times when I'm very frustrated and annoyed and I'm doing things because I should do them and they have to be done... and that's valid and I can talk that through and that's all right. But I recognise, in a sense, that I'm not by nature a carer, I don't think. I think I've been a good mother and I'm a careful person. I don't know what sort of mother I'd explain myself as, a bit spartan in a sense. I'm physically fairly loving to my kids and I've always been mentally challenging to them. I get on very well with my children and they love to be home and all of those things. But I don't think by nature I'm a carer. So to be the carer for my mother has been something that I've had to work at. I can manage it because there has to be all that thinking ahead and recognition that I need to have a meal for this and a something for that. And I've got to be conscious of checking where she's put things and has she got money. (21)*

Children and caring for the elderly

Almost half of our participants had dependent children still living at home. Children also need care and attention; they demand a lot of time and emotional energy. When women are working, looking after children and carrying a major responsibility of care for an elderly relative, it places considerable strain upon everyone in the family. We have written already of the stress experienced by the women in this situation. Children are also affected. Some of these impacts are generally positive or at least educational; others are certainly detrimental.

> *I probably think it's been hardest for my son. He was born when the other three grandparents had all died, whereas the other children have all known them. So he has only known my mother and he's really only known her since she's been with us and he has basically just seen this decline. I think that's very hard for him at times and although she loves him, if she's cross and snappy with any one, she's cross and snappy with him. I guess it's because he's little. It's that whole authority area. So he does occasionally get a bit of flack from her and he finds that hard. It would be impossible having her in the house with us. [Mother is accomodated in a mobile home in the backyard.] I think that that would be too destructive and we couldn't continue with that, but I think as it is he manages and in the long term, as I said, it won't be a bad thing for him. I'm just sad he hasn't had the other. But that's got nothing to do with this situation that's, just the reality of it. It certainly doesn't do children any harm to see that they can have a small role in caring and they do, they are very supportive. But I would hate them to feel like they had to be doing a major amount or that their life was being terribly dislocated and burdened by it. I don't think that's just to them. (21)*

There are no ready answers here. One thing however is clear. No one can carry on indefinitely in such situations without ongoing and reliable support. Nor can such caring loads be sustained unless there is relief and respite. And there are in the lives of all children points of crisis or periods when they have need of extra support and consideration, such as in the case of a serious accident or illness, sitting for the Higher School Certificate examination, major problems at school or with the police. Children need to have their parent's undivided attention at such times and, of course, those times are not always able to be predicted. Just knowing that if the need arises one can take that time and that, for a stretch, someone else will take over the "worrying" about ones elderly parents and their situation, would be a great relief and would lessen the strain of caring.

Men and caring

A number of the women reflected upon the issues of gender and caring. How the men in one's life respond to one's caring responsibilities is clearly of critical importance. This is true not just of the response of male partners and brothers, but also of male colleagues at work and male "bosses". Those women who commented on men and caring were, by and large, very critical of the men with whom they worked. There was also a great deal of frustration that so little had changed and despair that the gendered nature of caring remained so entrenched.

> *Yes I really do (think it would make a difference with a male boss). That's just coming from pure prejudice I suppose. Unless a male boss was in the situation where he had an aged relative and was really right there with you and empathising because he was in a similar situation, I'm sure he would be thinking of the pragmatic kind of facts of things rather than the situation. (29)*

> *I think it's very difficult for people with care responsibilities anyway... We take sick leave, when our kids are sick. Male colleagues don't do that. They will write on the white board, "Looking after children; not in for a week". We take sick leave ourselves. There's a gender difference there, clearly. We are so aware of having to do it all and not make too many demands on our employment. It's really hard. And it's been interesting in the last couple of years because several of my male colleagues have actually had care responsibilities with other children living with them or ageing parents living with them. Two of my colleagues at the moment are going through this experience and their behaviour towards me has changed... A real understanding, this is what it's like! I can't help but feel, for example, when (Mother-in-law) was living with us, I never took any sick leave. One of my colleagues whose mother is dying of a brain tumour at the moment, a male, he's virtually taken the last three months off and everyone's saying, poor (...), poor (...). I mean I wouldn't have done that and they probably wouldn't have said poor (...), poor (...), anyway. I don't think I'm being sexist or unfeeling of his situation, on the contrary. No, I just think that men get a lot more notice taken of their care responsibilities and their care needs. I mean we remark on the fact that the men, when we have staff meetings at 4.25, say, "Have to pick up the kids". Women always stay to the end. So I mean there's something going on there, which again isn't fair to women. (16)*

> *Particularly when women are often forced to work. Sometimes they want to work and that's great, but sometimes they are forced to work with large numbers of children and that's a strain. And they do all the housework when they come home because the husband doesn't really help and to be faced with the responsibility of being a carer, with say an Alzheimers parent, it's just too much to cope with. I think for a lot of those sorts of people, without those*

social supports, (it is an impossible situation). This business of caring has primarily been a women's issue and I think there is a whole, huge area to look at. Why women are willing to take this on and issues of duty and responsibility and those sorts of issues that quite often men don't feel. But I have to say in my husband's case he took on a lot of those issues. But I know for a lot of families and a lot of women I have in my carer's groups, it is the women who take on that role. On their own. Either we become, as the economic rationalists would have us become, very much a "user pays" society and it's a "me first" society and you don't show any sort of concern for your fellow human beings, or you start putting money where your mouth is. (4)

I'm fifty two. One of the arguments that you often see in the literature is just that just as women are getting to retirement age is the point at which their parents disintegrate and by the time they've got over caring for their parents in a sense they are too old to enjoy anything much themselves. I feel in some ways that is misguided in the sense that promotion normally comes later to women and if you are round about the end of your working life when the crisis comes it's also the point at which you are just beginning to be secure enough perhaps to stand on your rights and ask for the same treatment as men. So that's one thing. The other thing which I think I should emphasise is the fact that I found other women enormously supportive. Some of the men around here who have been through the same thing themselves have, in a sense, earned a certain amount of merit through doing that in a more public way, were also at least lip-service supportive and that was in some ways appreciated at the time too. I didn't actually have any men who were actively hostile to me doing that. (39)

Where male colleagues had been supportive it was almost always the case that they had had some similar caring experience. Yet the likelihood of a man actually having to care in the way that many women colleagues were caring was, in these working environments, very rare. As is evident elsewhere in this report, real, practical and sustained support from a male partner was not something that could be taken for granted and brothers were even less reliable.

Advice to other carers

As a result of their experiences of caring for and caring about an elderly relative, the women in this study had acquired a wealth of practical knowledge, skills and insights of a kind that were clearly of value to others. There was for some a reluctance to appear to presume to tell others, who might be in a rather different situation from their own, how to manage their lives. But if advice was simply a matter of sharing what they had discovered themselves through the experience, then they were more than ready to pass that on to anyone who was interested. If it helped another carer or helped ensure a better policy debate about the needs of carers, then that was a real bonus.

The advice ranged over a number of areas. Most immediate is the need to get as much help as you can. Carers need to find out as much as they can about the support services in their area, to talk to as many people as possible and then ensure they take advantage of what is on offer.

> *I think the first thing, I'd make sure that they had as much help as they could and I mean help, not just saying, "Oh yes, I'll be there to help". (3)*

> *Take full advantage (of) and find out everything that's going on in the welfare area. Find out what's going through a lot of the Community Options projects and a lot of the existing organisations. Also, if you've got aged relatives in hospitals, really get them to pick the social worker's brains to find out what's going that can help you. (29)*

Being aware of what is available was seen as crucial. Most of the women had little awareness of services, but also realised how important support services were. The advice offered was, don't be afraid to ask for help.

> *I think I might have done better if I'd asked more people earlier for information and each time it was a kind of reactive thing. If you see a crash coming, find out as much as you can from everybody. (39)*

> *Ringing up a disability service anywhere to get some information from. There is a group that can give you information on stroke patients. And then try to pin down (what needs to be done). The problem with care providers are (that) these nursing homes have a routine. There's no use speaking to specialists. They are a useless bunch. (38)*

And it wasn't just formal support services that were discussed. The importance of feeling able to call on the support of family and friends was also stressed.

> *If you have the option to prepare for it, to get your people on side now as in brothers and sisters, aunts, uncles, your children, friends, whoever. My advice would be if you know before it's going to happen, you know what's coming, try to prepare for it. Try to get your support group ready. That*

would be the smart way. It's called organisation. Plan for the future. Hopefully you can plan to get the support in line. Where possible, don't take it all on yourself. But if that's the case, if you plan for it or you've got really good friends who are willing to support, great, use them. But be careful on how much you use them depending on what your relationship is. (17)

Try and enlist as much help as you can from friends, neighbours, whoever is out there in the community. Use as many people as you can. (37)

Many stressed the importance of trying to establish limits, some understanding of what you can manage reasonably and where you think you're going to have to draw the line. Nevertheless establishing limits, although important, is not always so easily achieved.

Well I thought of some strategies which I haven't actually put into practice. I've thought of things like saying to Mum, "Every second weekend I will put aside a day for you but the other weekend I'm not coming". I haven't done it. I think one needs to do it from the outset. I suggest that people consider contracting for that sort of thing about recognising that you are going to need time where you don't feel guilty about the fact that you are not there. And if you can set the boundaries early it's much easier. (35)

As in the discussion of stress, the advice to others placed considerable emphasis on the importance of having time to yourself, of looking after yourself and your health, of having interests outside work and caring. Again there is the need to recognise the inherently stressful nature of what you are doing and thus the importance of not expecting too much of yourself nor hesitating to ask for help when you need it. Don't wait until you're going under, try and negotiate some time for yourself right from the start.

One has to be quite strong to make an effort to look after yourself. (35)

I would say find something (meditation) that gives you pleasure, takes you right out of yourself and the situation that you are in. Not that you want to escape necessarily, although in the first instance it was a means of escape, but find something that you yourself are interested in, that the person that you are looking after, can't necessarily be involved in. It needs to be something that you yourself are involved in. If you are in a caring role where you are more restrained than what I am at present, you need to have time to yourself, where you have one evening a week, a month, where it is just your time and you organise somebody else to look after that person for that time. You must have time to yourself. That would be the most important thing. (12)

You have to care for yourself because if you are not fit to look after them, who is going to look after them? You have to look after yourself first. So many people come through emergencies. "I can't come into hospital, who is going to look after my mother?" You can't look after your mother while you are ill. You need to get better so that you can look after her. Maybe your mother needs to look after you for a while. (19)

Love yourself, nurture yourself and then you can do that for others. (33)

Definitely make time for yourself. Don't feel guilty if you're going to make time for yourself. I think it's very important. You have to start thinking about yourself. Having outside interests is very, very important. Even doing relaxation and stress management courses and opening up to people who you can trust so you can air your problems and have that emotional support. I think that's very, very important. So you feel like someone's there supporting you emotionally - your partner or friend - making others aware that you're not a super mum or super person, that you've got your own needs, your own emotions, to deal with. (30)

One of the participants pointed to the need not to take the outbursts and behaviour of one's parent personally and to try and retain a sense of proportion in it all. Humour was an important component in dealing with the stress as was learning to stand up for yourself.

Try not to personalise outbursts and practices such as a person's behaviour in public. I still don't quite care to take Mum into a restaurant but I don't mind taking her to a cafe. Learn to laugh. Be open, be honest as much as you possibly can, be yourselves. Be as assertive as you possibly can with the person that you are caring for. (9)

Talking to as many people as possible in similar situations or working in community services, hospitals or aged care generally, was seen as vital. Carer support groups are important and other carers are a ready source of knowledge about what is available, about the pitfalls, about coping.

Just that it's good to have friends to talk to when you're making decisions about whether it should be a nursing home or care at home. And it's good to have friends who understand. I have a friend who's worked for many years with elderly people in nursing homes and I found it very helpful to be able to

> *talk to her. And also I think just that the frailty of your own parent is just an emotional reminder of how you might be at that stage of life and that part of you doesn't want it for yourself just as you don't want it for your parent. So you have to cope with your feelings about that. Sometimes you find you can talk to other people, like I can talk with this friend about that because she understands. Otherwise you keep these feelings inside yourself I think without seeing the possible future for yourself that you wouldn't chose. (1)*

> *I think it's very important to be able to sit down and talk over, reflect with people. I think people involved in a situation should be able to sit down and talk it through, without getting emotional. Just talk through these are the things, and this is what you are experiencing, to be able to say things and do things and talk about things without emotion and feelings of hurt or anything like that. Just to think about things. (20)*

Talking through the issues with one's partner and with others who are close to you and who are likely to be affected by the decision to take on a major responsibility of care, is also essential. Allow time for the other significant relationships in your life.

> *I think that for families, it has to be really agreed with the spouse, that you need to be able to talk to that spouse, maybe even before marriage. Because it could be his parents or relative that you are going to be caring for and have fairly good ideas of what's going to happen. (40)*

> *Your relationship, that's the most important part. If it's a father or mother or son or daughter, that you allow time for the relationship that you've got. If that falls apart, well everything else falls apart. (3)*

The relationship with the elderly relative will inevitably change and may well require a major adjustment or re-negotiating of the roles of daughter and parent. Accepting that and trying to deal with it in a careful, compassionate yet firm way, is difficult but very important.

> *The only advice I could give is to make sure that you learn that they reach a stage where you have to be the senior person, rather than them as the father they have been all our life. I just had to learn to realise that he was no longer in that position and that's a big factor of learning, I think. That was just my biggest hurdle with my father, to learn that instead of him being the one in control, I had to learn that I had to be his strength. A role reversal, the child becoming a parent. He then became more like a child, where he'd*

> *be terribly upset and terribly distressed (yet) in five minutes I can have him laughing and realise that you can't listen to what he has to say. Until I learned that, I struggled. I used to go home very upset because he was in such a state until I learned that you then had to train him, or change his life a bit. Now it's not a problem. (34)*

Other advice related to more practical matters such as living arrangements. In the case of co-residence, the need for a degree of privacy for both carer and parent was emphasised by a number of participants.

> *If living in the same household, try to ensure privacy, for the carer and the "caree". If you could possibly find in your own house, or build a granny flat or whatever, for them to have their own space, for privacy, if that was at all possible, I would say definitely, that's the preferred thing. (13)*

Keeping a journal and writing down what is happening and how you feel was also suggested.

> *For the first six months of this year I realised I was just talking at anyone who'd listen and just putting a totally unfair burden on my friends. I started writing it down in a diary and when I looked at it I realised the hidden resentment against certain people who were the unacknowledged audience of what I was writing and I realised I had this really big and totally unfair resentment against my sister. I realised that was really unfair and then I started to write it all down and resolve a lot of it in writing. Also it's amazing how much information you build up about their situation and their needs and how you can monitor them and how useful it was for doctors. Interestingly enough since the Home and Community Care people have been coming in once a week and my own dilemma has been resolved, I've stopped writing it all down. (31)*

The importance of trying to hold onto a sense of orderliness and maintain a balance in your life was noted. But it was also important to be ready to reschedule your goals and priorities when circumstances change. This should not mean giving up what have been important goals for you but accepting that they may need to be put to one side for the moment.

> *It's about knowing what's most important in your life, who are the most important people and it's about balance, it is about balance. (33)*

Several women spoke of the importance of valuing what you are doing and of learning to "roll with the punches". Situations change and in many ways it does become easier. Nevertheless, no one can hope to be "on top of things" all the time.

This sounds defeatist and I can see why a women would resent this resolution, but to roll with the punches and to be - it sounds as though you are saying cop out or give into it. I'm not prepared to give up my goals, but just to reschedule them. But that's really easy for me to say because I've got more education, more flexibility, more cultural capital, I'm more in control of my workplace than most women. Maybe just not to give up, not to give up your own educational and other goals, even if you have to shelve them (for the time being). (31)

All I can say is hang in there because it does improve. You think at the time that it's not going to, but it does improve. (25)

We just have to ride it. There's a lot of things in life you just have to ride and that's one of them. And how long do you really have your Mum or Dad? Even treat it as a precious time because it's a learning experience for the other members of the family. And I think family is such an important thing and even as old as they are it sort of gives a richness to the family. (41)

There is an end to the tunnel. That you do feel trapped sometimes but that there are other things out there and once that stage has passed that you can get on with your life. (40)

The virtues of patience and tolerance were extolled.

You have to have patience; you have to be able to understand. (2)

Be patient, be very understanding, put yourself in the other person's position and see what it's like. In a funny way be very grateful because as well as being under a lot of stress, under a lot of tension, aggravation, happiness, sadness, you are learning so much. You don't realise how much you are really learning. Everyday I learn, every day. (15)

Have a laugh, have a cry, a cup of tea, a Bex and a good lie down. (9)

And the most forthright and unequivocal advice of all.

I'd say, get out quick. (18)

The advice offered by our participants to others in similar situations reinforces most of the major findings of this study. Caring is not something which should be taken on lightly and is not a responsibility that any one person should carry on their own. As outlined above, the most frequently proffered advice was to organise as many supports and services as possible, drawing on family, friends, workmates and community resources. Our participants emphasised again and again the importance of both formal and informal support in caring for dependent relatives.

Another frequently repeated piece of advice was to look after yourself. Many of the women in this study had learnt this lesson the hard way and were anxious that other women not repeat their mistakes. Some of these stories are documented in the chapter on the stress of caring.

And lastly was the observation that things do change, that the actual crises are generally relatively short-lived, and although stressful and wearing don't constitute all that caring will mean. Life does regain some predictability and one does find one's self being able, most of the time, to manage with a degree of equanimity and to carry on caring.

For all the emphasis on the importance of self care, of valuing what you are doing, of the understanding and enrichment that may be gained from the experience of caring, there is also an acknowledgment that this is difficult and, at times, very stressful work. It is not for everyone. Some should probably not take on co-resident caring. And for those already caring at home, the time may come when some other arrangement for the care of one's parent should be made. For both those who are engaged in co-resident caring and those whose parents live separately, adequate respite and relief remain of vital importance.

Conclusion

We have included in this book a chapter devoted to reflections on caring and advice to other carers for two basic reasons. In the first place it was hoped that we might be able to provide carers and service providers, with some useful insights and some practical tips that might help improve the immediate circumstances of some carers or, at the very least, reassure people that their own experiences and responses are shared and understood by others. They are not alone or unique in finding the multiplicity of tasks involved in caring, and most of all the emotional load, difficult and stressful. Other chapters in the report reinforce this message.

The second reason was to try and draw out something of the essence of the experience of caring. It was felt that in reflecting and in giving advice, participants would be making their own assessment of what lay at the heart of things, of what were really the most important aspects, understandings, issues in caring for an elderly relative while working in the paid workforce.

What has emerged from this exercise is confirmation of what we have already tried to draw out of the accounts that form the basis for this research. Here it is in distilled form.

Caring is work and it is often arduous work.

Carers can only really continue to care if they are able to share the load and receive regular and reliable support.

Carers need to have time off, time to themselves. To be working full-time and caring the rest of the time, continuously, places unreasonable strains on the carer, her family and on the relationship with the elderly parent. Caring cannot be sustained in such circumstances, or at least, not for very long.

Caring for elderly parents is a worthy job and needs to be recognised for what it is, a contribution to the whole community as well as to the wellbeing of a particular individual. We all gain from the fact that people care. It is something which, as a community, we should be recognising and lauding. We need also to ensure that from this recognition flows concrete support.

8 Working Lives

For the women in this study, paid work was of considerable importance. This is hardly unexpected. While the accounts are particular and individual, of particular workplaces and of individual struggles to pursue a career and even, at times, to remain in work, the experiences are common. Very many Australian women including those who are not at present carrying a major responsibility of care, express similar views about the importance of work and face similar (although less extreme) difficulties in balancing the various demands in their lives. And while this report focuses on the attempt to juggle paid employment and unpaid caring work and the ambivalence and contradictions this creates for the women in this situation, it is important to acknowledge the wider political, economic and historical context in which such experiences take place, a context which reflects and, indeed, perpetuates conditions of greater vulnerability for women, in general, in the paid workforce.

Certain features of that wider context stand out. The fact that paid work is now a significant part of the lives of most women is the most obvious feature. Overall, the movement of women, particularly married women, into the paid workforce over the last twenty years, represents a radical social change. In the mid sixties, only 20% of married women were in paid work. Now it is more than 50% and rising. This increase has had a marked impact on women, on families, on the workplace and on community attitudes and values (Probert 1997). Home prices, rents and other basic commodities have risen and many households now need two incomes to live comfortably. And if the trend continues, and more and more women move into the workforce, the numbers of women who are both working and carrying some responsibility for the care of ageing relatives is likely to increase and increase substantially.

There is evidence that although women are participating more and more in the labour market, their earnings remain at a lower level than those of men. The majority of part-time workers are women and only a small proportion of women workers have had access to superannuation schemes. The position of women workers in the labour market is, in general terms, a relatively vulnerable one and women continue to be subject to pressures to move in and out of paid work depending on their caring responsibilities (Ibid., Bryson 1995a).

It has been argued that "full-year, full-time work is the best defence against poverty" (Cass 1985, quoted in Bryson 1992, p.206). Indeed, recent government policy initiatives have been aimed at alleviating the effects of unemployment by targeting groups that are seen to be particularly vulnerable to long term unemployment, such as sole parents (Bryson 1995b, p.69).

It is difficult to estimate the numbers of women who have withdrawn from the labour market to care. Stehlik, has pulled together the available statistics and argues that, "Although the data is not clear, the Australian Bureau of Statistics shows that in the twelve months prior to April, 1988, of the people who had left the labour force in the previous 12 months, 364,100 or 69% were women and more than 50% of these women were in the 25-44 year age group... Some 13.1% of women gave as their reason for ceasing their last job to look after family, house or someone else and of these, 4.5% said they intended not to return". Stehlik also refers to some of the earlier attempts to examine the impact of caring on paid work and the ability to continue to work full-time. She lists the 1983 study by Kinnear and Graycar which found that over 50% of carers gave up work in order to care, an Australian Council of the Ageing (ACOTA) survey published in 1986 which found that 11.2% gave up full-time work and research by Kendig and colleagues in 1983 which found that over 71% of their carers were not employed full-time (Stehlik 1993, p.17).

The women we interviewed were selected because they were both working full-time and carrying a major responsibility of care for an elderly relative. As stated earlier, we made use of a broad definition of "a major caring responsibility". We had a select group of workers who were trying to negotiate the demands of paid and unpaid work. They form, of course, a very small group and we make no claim that they are representative of even this category of carers. Nevertheless, there are recurring themes within this study that suggest common features of the experience of working and caring. In addition, the picture of care which emerges is consistent with that drawn in other studies of the caring experience. What is demonstrated in this research is that to work and care tends to exacerbate problems with both the caring role and the role of worker or, at least, bring them into sharper relief. At the same time, other features of the caring role such as isolation, financial insecurity and lack of any outlet, are, not surprisingly, less marked among those carers who were in paid employment.

For most of the women in this study, participation in the paid workforce was a given and non-negotiable part of their lives. The majority of them had no intention of giving up work at this stage. They were more than aware that moving in and out of the workforce at this stage of their lives was probably not a viable option. There are very good reasons for holding onto your job if withdrawal from the workforce means dependence on social security in the short term and, given that the chances of re-entry in the future are slight, in the long term as well. For many of the women in this study, choosing to give up their jobs to care full-time for their relatives would be a route to poverty in their own old age.

The income from paid work was essential for the majority of these women. They worked to support themselves and their families. Some were single women. Several others were sole income earners. So, financial considerations were uppermost. For these women there was no real choice. There was a clear recognition that labour market participation was important for their survival. With only one exception, all the women had been in the paid workforce for some time before they had taken on major caring responsibilities. They had entered the labour force with the expectation that they would work until retirement.

In addition, work was an important part of their lives, of who they were. This, too, is borne out in other studies (Glezer & Wolcott 1997, p.29). Most of our participants enjoyed the work they were doing; some were quite passionate about their jobs. Involvement in paid work and all that comes with that - financial independence, job satisfaction and enjoyment - was also an important part of their picture of themselves.

"I couldn't give up work"

> *I couldn't do it. (Give up work to care full-time.) Financially there's no way I could even consider it. (30)*

Some of the women had husbands or partners who were unemployed or retired, or had low incomes or irregular employment.

> *No, it's not an option because we can't afford to. I want to earn my own money and it's mine, which carries on from my family tradition, I suppose. I don't like being dependent. My husband is the main provider but I like to feel that I'm bringing in some money. So, no it's not an option. Probably not an option for my relationship either because my husband says that I'm really boring when I'm not working because I ask him too many questions about his work. (36)*

Another consideration that was mentioned was the cost of caring for a dependent person. Caring for someone at home can be an expensive undertaking. One women described this as an added reason for holding onto her job.

I had to try and keep working at the time. We had to pay to have the house modified: we had to pay for a wheelchair: we had to pay for a special chair, because he can't use an ordinary chair. All these things had to be paid for. So I had to try and keep working to keep that going. (25)

One woman had taken up paid work when her father moved into a nursing home to assist with nursing home expenses.

I started working really to keep up Dad's payments in the nursing home. That was really why I went back to work. I was free to have a part-time job and it wasn't fair on my husband's money to cope with the extra amount. We all shared in his costs at the time. So it was because of my father. That was originally why I started coming back to work. (34)

"I go to work for a holiday"

Work was valued for other reasons. Many women mentioned the enjoyment and satisfaction they gained from their jobs. They liked working, felt they were good at their jobs and were making an important contribution through their work.

Yes. I enjoy working, don't get me wrong, I love doing my work and there's no way I'm going to give it up. I'd go batty being at home seven days a week; that's not my cup of tea. But what time I do have at home, I like to enjoy and relax and it's not possible. I don't want to give up my weekend job because I want to do so many things and you have to have money to do all these wonderful things and I'm not a person that has credit cards and charges things. (3)

I've often said this job was made for me: this is it. I love talking to people and the people in this industry are really caring lovely people. It's just nice: it's another interest. If I was home with her all the time, it would be really boring, because she's got no conversation. (13)

One woman spoke with warmth of her workplace.

I'm very happy here, it's like my second home. (24)

And for another woman...

Work is my life. (39)

A number of women commented on the different nature of their paid work and their unpaid work and the different needs their paid work fulfilled. For some of the women their jobs provided them with fulfilment that was not generally present in their role as carers.

> *I'd love to give up work, but then I keep thinking, it's my outlet. I need a certain amount of work to get me away from the home environment. Sometimes I go there (to work) with great relief. (17)*

> *I would go spare if I stayed at home. I had time off when I had the children, but once they went to school, I came back to the workplace. I'm not the sort of person who doesn't work. I don't think very many women are these days. (25)*

> *In a funny sense it helps keep you sane, because it is something you are doing for yourself. You are not just doing it for the money. Everyone that works there loves what they are doing. (15)*

> *When I get there, I'm another person. I just carry on and forget all about this family. (6)*

And most telling of all...

> *I go to work for a holiday. (42)*

The majority of our participants were unable or unwilling to give up paid work, even if their circumstances changed. They would consider other options first, and hoped they would not have to make this decision. The ambivalence they felt was clearly expressed. They would like to continue work; they would have to continue to work. If their elderly parent needed more care, they might withdraw from the workforce, but for most it would be a very difficult decision to make. There are two apparently conflicting demands and rights. On the one hand, is the obligation to care and the belief in the right of those in your care to have the greatest quality of life it is in your power to provide. On the other hand, there is your own right to income security now and in the future and your entitlement to have rewarding work. This is the perennial dilemma which confronts the carer who works.

> *It is an extremely difficult question. By choice I'd rather continue working and cope with whatever I have to cope with. If it meant the quality of my mother's life is depleted, well, then I'd be forced into making a decision.*

Nothing is more important than family and quality time with her is very important. But I'd be looking at all the options. (33)

One said she would stop working if she had to, but that it would be,

Against my will. (31)

Despite a reluctance to give up work, some acknowledged that they may have to re-think this position in the future. Most stressed they would consider other options, depending on what the future held.

I don't want to give up work at this stage and I don't want to change. I like what I do. I certainly wouldn't want to go anywhere else, but I think if it came to the stage, that Mum needs a little bit more care I probably would either do less hours at work, or perhaps short-term take time off work, without pay, to see how it worked out. I wouldn't leave and then make a decision, because I might make the decision to go and then Mum may go to a nursing home or it may not work out or she may pass away. This is very evident in the Carer's Association. I've been going to all these seminars and conferences about what does the carer do when the lifeline goes? So I wouldn't say I would give up work tomorrow. I would ask for leave without pay. (2)

One woman was clear about the choice she would make.

I'd leave work. My mother comes first. (11)

Another women expressed how torn she felt in having to make such choices.

Guilt is the biggest thing. There's every part of me that is saddened every day because of that guilt and it sits very heavily with me. (22)

One of the questions asked was whether there had been any pressure exerted by those around them for them to give up their paid work. For most of the women this was not a major issue. There were, however, a few exceptions. Some of the elderly parents were not happy about their daughters continuing to work. There appeared to be a general lack of understanding of the important part that work played in the lives of their daughters. Perhaps this was because these parents belonged to a generation when it was uncommon for women to work after marriage and they saw work as an optional extra that could be shelved if necessary.

> *I guess I feel a certain resentment about the expectation she has of me and the comments she makes like, "There's no need for you to work. It's just that younger people these days are very greedy and want much more than we ever had when we were bringing up a family". Those sorts of comments, made me a bit angry, I think. She has actually suggested that I give up work and care for her. (35)*

However, in most of the accounts we collected there was simply no expectation on the part of the elderly person that the carer give up her job: it was just never considered an option.

> *I don't think mum would expect that from me or any other child. She knows that we need to work. An income has to come in. (23)*

One woman felt that her mother would actually be very upset if she realised her daughter had even contemplated giving up her job.

> *In fact, I kept on working because I thought if Mum ever gets better she'd be devastated if she knew what I'd done. (36)*

One of the participants reflected on the class issues involved in any consideration of women and work and family responsibilities.

> *I think the issues to do with work for women are often issues for middle class women. I think for a lot of working class women there's no quality of life in work. You're working in a factory. It's the pits. If you are a nice middle class woman with an education and you know the advantages in society, someone like me, I like going to work. But I grew up in a working class family; my father was a truck driver, my mother worked in a pencil factory. For both of them, work wasn't that good. It was an economic necessity to feed the kids and pay the bills. I think it's useful to look at work from a class perspective in some respects because sometimes it's not all it's made out to be. (4)*

This is an important reminder that class issues, financial status and, one must add, race and ethnicity, must be part of the equation. We cannot, must not, disregard these questions. They are critical both in relation to employment and caring and the relationship between them.

Impact of caring on working life and career

The complexities and contradictions inherent in juggling work and family lives were highlighted in the discussions focusing on the impact of caring responsibilities on working lives and career prospects.

The question asked was, "How has caring affected your working life"? Assessing the extent of this impact was sometimes difficult. Most of the women felt that their caring responsibilities had affected their working lives and their career progression in quite tangible ways, although there was a tendency to understate or play down the influence of the one upon the other.

Setting priorities

Although, in general terms, work was a given, the overwhelming pattern that emerged in the women's responses was an emphasis on "prioritising", a continual process of making decisions about what was most important to them at that time. For the majority, their career or "getting ahead" in their job, was not and could not be a top priority for the time being.

> *My career comes at the bottom of the list. It's something that I dearly want to do, but I can't because of all the dependants I've got around me. (41)*

Some women qualified this particular ordering of priorities by saying they'd pick up their careers later.

> *It's not the end of the world; it happens to everybody and I feel confident that in the future I will have a career again. (36)*

The time they devoted to caring was taken from other parts of their lives or had meant giving up other activities. In general the women played down the significance of these decisions and the impact they had had both on their work and their leisure. Time taken from work, especially a decision to cut back on hours for any extended period, was much less likely than simply a decision to "stay put" or to accept that they were "marking time" in their careers. Their career progression was "put on hold" for the time being. They were prepared to continue with the work they were doing but felt unable or unwilling to put energy into furthering their careers, applying for promotion or changing jobs.

For many of the women it was further education and training and upgrading their qualifications that were shelved or sacrificed. Others had deliberately chosen to change jobs and sought employment in an area where they knew they would have more flexibility and therefore be able to continue in the paid workforce, while continuing to carry fairly onerous caring responsibilities.

Making work manageable

For some of the women, the decision to postpone or not participate in part-time study or training programs that would formally upgrade their skills and qualifications was clearly a significant, self-imposed limitation on future career progression and choice. It has meant cutting off the possibility of more rewarding or better paid or simply different work at least for the time being.

A number spoke of how they had given brief consideration to the pursuit of further qualifications but quickly realised the futility of taking on an extra load at this point in their lives.

> *I'd like to study, I really would, but I'm afraid I can't have my job, look after my Mother, study. I can't have everything in life. That's one thing which is very unlikely that I will go on (with). But you never know may be something could come up. (11)*

> *I'd love to go on and do further training courses at night and weekends which I can't. Caring has interfered there. I've had to give up my "Lifeline" work; I can no longer do that. Nor participate in on-going education, the workshops and things of that nature which were very helpful. (37)*

> *I couldn't continue tertiary education. When degrees were being offered and we could take credits for being a RN (registered nurse). I was only forty and I worked out where a lot of the girls around my age were starting it. I knew that I couldn't cope. It was too much of a burden for me to cope, because I've also got an eighty two year old Mother-in-law living beside me. So my responsibilities were just too high. (10)*

> *I would quite like to have done some further study at this point, I just don't have the energy to do that because weekends I also usually give her one day at the weekend, whether it be going and getting her and washing her hair or doing the washing, taking her for a drive or just having her at home. (35)*

For those women working in universities, placing further study "on hold" had dramatic implications for their future careers, putting them out of the running for jobs in the university, or condemning them to the secondary labour market of casual, part-time tutoring, low paid, uncertain and without continuity of employment.

> *I probably should say that the prospect of finishing my PhD is at risk. And, if it is, my future employment is at risk - either casual teaching or, at the best, hanging in as a tutor. (31)*

> *Well I started my Masters and in April just decided I had to give it away. Something had to go. That costs me money, it doesn't earn me any. My contract has expired for the second time so I had to reapply here and I think my chances are - I mean I've got an interview - but I think my chances are very slim really because of my academic qualifications. I've certainly given all to my teaching, but as you would know, in academia you need to keep your studies up. (36)*

Or for others, it was a matter of caring responsibilities precluding any possibility of a career change.

> *Well I guess I now see the job that I'm in will be the job that I will remain in until I choose to stop work. Then I will do some of those things that I might have actually made a new career, as purely an interest thing. (35)*

Other strategies that were adopted included putting their career progression "on hold", withdrawal from promotion or advancement for the time being. In some cases participants had refused promotion and chosen to work in the locality that was in close proximity to the dependant they were caring for.

> *I chose to compromise my career for bringing up my children. My children always came first while they were in need of my care. Now that they've grown up and gone I should be able to put more energy into my career. It's more demanding and I also would like to be able to meet those demands to give me a feeling, before I end my working life, that I've given it all I can, which I feel I didn't necessarily do when the kids were younger. And I now feel I can't because of the demands of Mum. (35)*

> *I would really like to go for promotion, but I feel that while I'm so stretched I'm not prepared to take on the administrative work. It's not something I have the energy for at the moment. Maybe in five years time. (16)*

> *I think it has restricted me in(terms of) where I've worked. As far as location (is concerned), not so much in career direction. I've kept my goals in that*

area, but have been disappointed in that I haven't done more travel and worked in more places than I have. (19)

Some participants had deliberately chosen to work in jobs where they had more control over their time, jobs with more flexibility. One woman related the story of how she felt she was "lucky" that she had been a full-time student when her mother became ill.

I might say that it was lucky for me that I had become a full-time student at the time when Mum demented. If I had have been in full-time paid employment I'd be in absolute crisis now. So it was just really lucky that I was able to pick up more flexible work patterns. (31)

This woman mentioned how her actual choice of career had been affected as a result of the experience of caring for her mother.

I find that I haven't got a high geriatric tolerance. It definitely has classified my level of nursing. I did nurse in a nursing home. I found it frustrating because it was a sort of terminal type nursing, but that was initially before I even came here. When I came here I did some medical nursing but found it wasn't my forte. I wanted more acute care, and people who actually got better and went home. I found that I could deal with speed, I could deal with complications, but I couldn't deal with the on-going geriatric demands. I just felt that I wasn't a geriatric nurse any more. My tolerance was lowered with the persistence of coping with my Mother. I found nursing, coming here, an outlet. I couldn't possibly stay at home and cope with her constantly. I had to have an outlet. My colleagues here helped me a lot. If I get a geriatric patient and I find my tolerance is lowering, they'll take over for me, because they are able to appreciate, so I find them a great help. (10)

Another commented on the fact that she had progressed to a stage in her working life that better accommodated her caring responsibilities than the previous positions she had held.

I have a management kind of role now rather than a direct social work role and it's got it's own particular difficulties about it but it's not as emotionally draining as some of the social work I've done in the past. For instance, I worked in the admission centre at... Hospital for a couple of years and I certainly wouldn't want to be doing that kind of work at this stage of life when emotionally perhaps my resources aren't as good as they were when I was younger. (1)

A few played down or dismissed the notion that their caring responsibilities had dramatically impacted on their working lives. They described making particular adjustments and choosing particular options but did not feel that they had been especially disadvantaged in their careers.

> *That doesn't mean I necessarily feel my career has been set back, it's been different. I checked every option and basically did the best thing for me while doing this. (39)*

Negotiating day by day: support in the workplace

One of the main concerns of this study was to explore what the women themselves felt were the factors that most enabled them to cope with their busy lives and multiple responsibilities. A major focus was the extent and nature of support and understanding they received in their paid work. Did they think there was an organisational culture supportive of those with family caring responsibilities? Were managers and colleagues understanding and informed about the issues involved? What were the factors in the workplace that alleviated or exacerbated the stress and anxiety of combining work and family responsibilities? Were there opportunities, for example, for negotiating on a day-by-day basis in these workplaces?

Some workplaces were clearly more congenial and open to the possibility of negotiation than others and there were particular features in several workplaces that had helped alleviate some of the difficulties the women were facing. In particular instances this had meant that the women were actually able to continue working where this would otherwise have been impossible.

This did not, however, occur in all the workplaces or even most that are reported on by our participants. At the other extreme, were workplace environments that were rigid, impersonal and difficult and where negotiation was impossible. As argued elsewhere, these situations exacerbated and added to the women's anxiety and stress levels.

When we asked whether there were aspects of the workplace that they felt made a difference to the ways in which were able to organise their lives, some of the women spoke of there being a supportive "culture" in their workplace, a culture that valued people's contributions and emphasised the importance of understanding workers' needs.

Some argued that perhaps this "understanding" environment could in part be explained by the type of work they did...

I think it's the organisation as a whole. I think because we do the sort of work we do, we're understanding of people in that sort of situation. My own work and (knowledge of) the resources... was very helpful with my own husband. I knew where to go and get things. I knew how to go and get them and that was great. My own job has been a big support in more ways than one. (25)

Or because of the kind of staff who typically choose to work in community services or in the welfare and health sectors.

Mind you the office is staffed by ninety percent women and there's only a couple of male managers in Homecare and this branch has always had a female manager. At the moment, both managers, this one and the one before, have been in similar situations to me and I guess most of us know that it could be us. So being women in similar situations they would be loathe to say, "No, you can't go", and have to put it down to the line of your job or your family. So we all co-operate and everybody's got a welfare consciousness anyway or they wouldn't be working here. (29)

Another factor that was mentioned frequently was the attitude of the supervisor or the person in charge. An understanding and supportive boss was mentioned by many of the women as alleviating stress and making it easier to cope with the competing demands of work and caring responsibilities.

I think that we are fairly lucky with our supervisor being sympathetic. It is a good place to work. (8)

I guess in my case I haven't a great deal to complain about. I've got a very supportive hierarchy and a lot of autonomy. (9)

A few commented on the fact that they had only had to deal with women supervisors or that their experiences with male and female "bosses" had been very different.

My boss was a really beaut example of a woman who knew, who understood, and made me feel really good about doing it, not a burden. She was pretty rare. The women were always very supportive. We had at that time a woman who was Head of Department, who knew our situation well and was magnificent. She would help me when I was feeling down; she would help me theorise it so I wouldn't personalise it. She was great at problem solving. So every time I saw her I would come away feeling marvellous, really empowered. With two male bosses it's been much less satisfactory, because they haven't had the experience basically or they don't want to know, I suppose. (16)

I've been very lucky in the last few years, I've had bosses that have been understanding and realised that if I have to go, I have to go. All my employers have been fully aware that my family comes first and that's the way it's always been, and they've been understanding. But I've never had a male boss. They've all been females. (19)

Others commented on the special qualities of a male supervisor.

As a person you can't fault him because he is really good, compassionate and he does think of his staff. He's stuck by me and helped me out when I've needed help. When he's seen me falling apart at the seams, he's just called me to the office and said, "Oh we're going to have to do something for you to help you get things sorted". He's really stuck by me during those years. (3)

A number of the participants in the study were managers themselves and recognised the importance of supporting their employees. They were genuinely interested in staff wellbeing. One manager commented on these issues at a number of points in the interview.

When my mother had her triple by-pass operation, I'd only been working here probably six months at the time and I've got to say the management and staff here were just very supportive. I think I learned myself many years ago in the workforce that if you look after your staff then they look after you as far as giving of their best when they can and I would expect with any of my staff if there's any sort of family problems I'm very quick to insist they have time off and to support them through that because the end product is a happy working place and people will cope because they're got that sort of backup. We here are part of (a larger organisation) so although I'm manager here my management comes from our head office and they are always very supportive and again they would be quick to almost insist that I had time off if I needed it and be flexible. (33)

Another woman made the point that experienced and skilled workers are worth holding onto.

Your biggest asset is your human resource and without your human resources, you're done. (17)

Not surprisingly, working in an understanding and supportive environment made a very real difference to those women fortunate enough to be in such a workplace. This understanding was generally followed by some tangible support and strategies designed to assist and support the women.

One of the ways managers assisted and supported employees was through the adoption of flexible working hours. In some workplaces this allowed the employee to work hours that fitted in, to some extent at least, with their caring responsibilities.

> *The biggest asset for me is the flexi-time, and our definition here of flexi-time is not that we can work any hours we want, we have to start and finish within certain times, but we can save up any overtime we do (rather than getting paid) and can take that time off when it suits us and the organisation. So, if you've got some time up your sleeve in the form of flexi time that's helpful. If I knew I needed to go for half a day somewhere with Mum, I'd could be pretty sure that I'll have some time that I can take off. Just having that flexibility in working hours is really helpful... I haven't got total freedom to work whenever I want, but just that little bit of flexibility is all I've needed up to now. I would imagine, however, that in a more difficult situation, if you had other family as well, it might need to be a bit more flexible. (29)*

One of the participants commented that she felt guilty about the amount of time she took off work.

> *Sometimes I get too much time and feel a bit guilty about my job. (7)*

In a number of cases negotiation was conducted between workmates. Being able to count on and negotiate with one's colleagues and workmates was often critical in managing the complex array of demands. Strategies adopted included covering for each other and swapping shifts.

> *This place obviously has to have twenty four hour coverage of staff. We're very quick to swap and change and have a few days off here and make it up there. Obviously some people don't want to take leave as such, but we do a lot of flexible compromising. (27)*

> *We have very flexible working arrangements. I think actually women's ways of working are quite finely honed. We support each other, for example. When someone's kid is sick we meet at their place. When someone's father is ill, we reschedule the meeting. We do things by 'phone and fax when someone is unable to come. So we actually work in a networking sort of way.*

So, I don't feel like I'm letting my colleagues down, because there's a mutuality about it. (16)

Workmates and colleagues also provided a "sounding board" and advice and moral support when circumstances were difficult.

I suppose I can come to work and air a lot of my problems. They probably think here she is talking about her mother again, but it's quite useful for me because I can talk about it and they'll either sympathise or suggest different strategies... If you're emotionally involved with someone, it's very hard and having three generations living in the house is difficult. I think most of the women are quite supportive. I'm not saying that (husband) isn't, because I wouldn't talk about those things to (husband) any way. (30)

My colleagues just keep me buoyant in terms of asking about me. It's just been on a one to one basis. It was mostly my soulmates on the staff who looked after me. (22)

There have been occasions where I've been really touched by the support that they've given me. Earlier this year I went through about a week where I was so emotional because I felt that I might only have Mum a month, so consequently I was very emotional and just out of the blue one day I came back from lunch and I'd been crying in the morning and there was a little spray of orchids, and one of the girls had got on the computer and done a graphic of a butterfly and put we care about you on the bottom of it, and it was just really special to think they felt that way. (12)

The support from others also took the form of sharing information and gleaning useful knowledge from those who had faced similar difficulties.

The support that you got mostly was through talking to other staff members and discussing. A lot of them had similar situations or knew of people getting help. Something like getting the power of attorney for my father and that again was in a practical nature. When I was having problems with the one home that he was in, I didn't feel he was being cared for properly and again I wasn't aware of how people were transferred and Deputy Matron assisted me in transferring my father to a nursing home closer to my home, one that they knew quite well, where he got excellent care. (40)

"I've had mixed reactions"

Not all employers were supportive. Where there was little support, the situations ranged from cases where the employers were oblivious to the fact that their employees were under any strain, to situations where the women's motives and behaviour were misinterpreted. The responses of employers and fellow workers ranged from decidedly negative, even obstructive, to hurtful, to unhelpful or simply a rather limited tolerance.

The less extreme or the oblivious...

I think they are probably more aware of the needs of staff who have children. (1)

I've had mixed reactions. There was a day here not so long ago when I spoke to Mum on the phone as a normal routine call and she sounded as though something was wrong and after a bit of questioning and ringing back again in a few minutes, I felt that she'd possibly had a slight stroke so I just had to tear out of the office and go. People were supportive, I guess, although that isn't the word that springs to mind. They were not obstructive and certainly didn't make it difficult for me, but everybody is just really busy here and gets on with their own thing. One colleague rang me at home to see that everything was okay. They weren't overtly supportive, but they weren't obstructive either. (29)

The negative, hurtful and unhelpful...

They were extremely inflexible in terms of deadlines. At one stage when they tell me, my father was unconscious at that stage they tell me I had to get my marks in by 9am on a given morning and then I found out this was so that person could have two days in which to enter the marks in the computer. If the marks had been another day late, by which time perhaps my problem would have been resolved once and for all. They could have been a bit more flexible there. (39)

The only time that was really a crisis actually was at the very end when he was very sick and it happened to be Easter and I got a negative response. It was from the nursing home and I think it was because it was Easter and I'd said that he was ill and actually he died that weekend, we didn't know that he was that ill. I just got a feeling of, "Oh, this is a fast one. You want the day off". So although the nursing home situation was good for support that way, they weren't very understanding generally. You had a duty to perform and you were expected to be there and you could sort your other problems, or somebody else could handle them. (40)

I had some trouble at work last year. I've never got over that and so I suppose the stress, is because I don't trust people anymore and I think that adds to the stress at home... I wouldn't think that its a very supportive environment at all. (20)

When it first came, the big crunch, we didn't know whether she was going to live or die. There was one particular night the doctors said she could go at any time, her blood pressure dropped, they couldn't even read it. I sort of tried to hold it in check at work. My boss caught me out and said, "Have you been out for a party or something", because my eyes were bulging out of my head from crying. For the first few weeks she was fine, everything was fine. She could understand there was an illness and that you were worried but it started to wear off. She started to think, "I realise she is ill but your not paying attention to work". So the pressure started to be on. Workwise it is still. I'd already had a couple of days when I moved house, or it was leave without pay, then I'm off for a couple of days, because when it first happened then because of all the running around, the stress involved, I wasn't eating, I wasn't sleeping properly. I could hardly perform...I wasn't performing well at work. I was also running myself down so I was having a couple of days off because I just couldn't move. I think they tended to think I was playing around. My boss calls me into the office and then starts to give me a dressing down and a formal written warning which goes on your file. Nowhere was there any room for me to comment, to say I thoroughly understand your situation however, there's a bit more to mine. There was really no great leeway. So I snapped. I thought if that's the way you want it to be, I'll play along with it. So from that point in time I kept my emotions very much in check and I found that at my particular place of work I've had to play a dual game. I go into work and I'm a total different personality. I act the fool, I get my work done and people think everything's dandy. But there's been no give and take so in terms of getting the response from work, the immediate boss is not particularly sympathetic and has been quite critical. (17)

There were cases where the women had been unable to take leave.

I actually went to social work department and asked if I could somehow take time off work. At this stage my mum wasn't in the hostel, she was still caring for herself. I asked could I take time off work and get some sort of a carer's pension but not actually leave my job, and I couldn't because even if I would

> *have taken leave without pay, I wasn't entitled to any benefit whatsoever, so I had to put her in a nursing home. (8)*

In a good many work situations the attitude was clearly that these difficulties were not the employer's problem. Some employers had known the situation their employees were in and yet had made unreasonable demands, had set deadlines that were unnecessary and unrealistic and had refused to grant leave in an emergency.

Another feature that emerged was that the women themselves tended to "downplay" the difficulties they were facing. In addition, when it came to asking for or negotiating varied working conditions, it was clear that there was an overall reluctance to ask for time off or, indeed, any concessions, let alone special provisions.

In some respects they placed the onus on themselves as workers, rather than the employer. In most cases this was reflected in the recurring emphasis on the attempt to keep work and family separate. However, a couple of our participants argued it was the carer's responsibility to inform the employer of her situation. One women had actually done this when she was interviewed for a job, and only accepted the job on the condition that the employer was aware of the responsibilities the carer was carrying and the possibility that she may require time off to deal with emergencies. Others made more general comments.

> *I think that's partly the carer's responsibility to let the employer know the situation. You have to communicate with the employer, so the boss can understand, because if you don't communicate, you've got the problem. They are not psychic, they can't understand. (12)*

> *Be understanding I think, but then a lot of that responsibility comes back on the carer. You need to be able to tell people what's going on. A lot of employers, I'd say, are ignorant of their employee's home situations until it gets to a crisis point. I made an issue when I was employed to discuss that my family situation was such that I just had to drop things and go, discussing that at the time of my interview and giving the employer a fair go to see whether they wanted to take that responsibility on when they employed me and I think the communications pathway between employer and employee need to be very open and there's a problem with that. And I think nine out of ten people are fairly understanding when it comes to issues like that. Flexibility comes in there. (19)*

There is little doubt that negotiating work and family responsibilities is a daunting task. However, there were clearly certain factors that made a tremendous difference to the ways in which these responsibilities were negotiated.

In those instances where there was some recognition of the responsibility the women were carrying and indeed that these responsibility were important and legitimate, there was room to negotiate and some of the employers were understanding and supportive of their employees. This resulted in the retention of valued, experienced and loyal workers. There was a recognition of the fact that these women were valued workers who deserved and merited the employer's support, and some of the employers were prepared to offer this "space". General acceptance of the legitimacy of family responsibilities, however, is still a long way off.

> *There's no leave for stress related things at all. There used to be, I think, and they scrubbed that from the policy... If people have family sick and they don't have leave owing, then they either take sick leave and pretend that they are sick, or just hope that whoever is in charge on the day is going to be good about it. I think so far that's been everybody's experience, but it is only the luck of the draw. (29)*

Accommodating needs: creating the "carer friendly" workplace

A major concern of this research has been to explore ways in which the workplace might be made to be more responsive to the particular needs of those juggling the competing demands of employment and unpaid caring work. We asked our participants what specific recommendations would they make for changes in the workplace so that these demands might be more easily managed and a little less stressful. Participants made a number of suggestions about how employers and others in the workplace could support those workers with family responsibilities, most particularly those caring for the elderly. The suggestions proposed are remarkably modest.

"Understanding" in the workplace

Most of the women said that what they really wanted was a recognition that those caring for elderly relatives had competing obligations, to their families as well as to their work. Allied with this recognition was the hope that there would also be an acknowledgment from employers and fellow workers that fulfilling one's family responsibilities was an important and legitimate activity. So, top of the list of ways to improve their own working lives and the lives of those in similar situations was a call for more understanding.

> *I think that if they listen to women who have had this experience, just listen. (36).*

> *Just be understanding I suppose. (13)*

One woman drew on her own experience and used as an example the way her own employer had behaved during the time she was burdened with particularly onerous caring responsibilities.

> *I think that employers could do what my employer did. They knew the situation, they knew the problems and accepted that it was going to get better, it's not going to get worse. He did improve from the stroke, so things have got easier for me and I'm coping better. (25)*

> *Understand that women have many roles and many responsibilities and support them. I think maybe if they had more of a background file, not getting too personal, but understanding. Most people don't know anything about the other person and so if they develop a personnel file, letting women know that if you need that time, yes, that's fine. Or if you need some counselling, maybe if they could put them in the right direction and personnel officers often can do that. Being flexible. (40)*

> *Just understanding from the workplace that leaving elderly and vulnerable people at home on their own for long periods until you return is bad form. (16)*

> *I can't think of anything except for it to be okay to not feel guilt if you are looking after a parent. For somebody in the workplace to say we understand this, we know that it is a long term thing. It may mean that your career has to take a different path, but how can we help? How can we adjust things so that you are not feeling that you are not giving it your best? (36)*

It was argued that alongside this understanding should come the recognition and acknowledgment that time taken up caring for an elderly relative is a legitimate and important activity.

> *Much the same I suppose they are being forced to acknowledge the needs of child care. The government is not going to support people in nursing homes*

> *and those sort of institutions. Basically it will be individuals that are going to have to support their elderly relatives and wanting and needing to be in the workforce. (9)*

> *I think that one of the important things is that you write on a CV (curriculum vitae, i.e., document setting out one's qualifications and employment record) that you've had time off due to family commitments and that it is taken very seriously. (36)*

Another woman felt that going through the experience was the only way to ensure that managers understood.

> *The only way they can support it, is they have gone through it themselves, but if they haven't experienced that and if the employer is a younger person, who hasn't had that experience, I think they should be more aware of what is really happening. (It's) only people in my age group that are going through it (that) can be (truly) understanding. (41)*

One participant felt that keeping her problems to herself and exhibiting an outward ability to cope when her world was falling apart, was perhaps not the most constructive way forward.

> *A lot of it's education I suppose. It could be my fault because I'm not one to go in there and talk to them and sit down and have a cry. I tend to say, "Well, I've got to bear it all, it's my problem, I've got to deal with it" and I know that's wrong. You should be able to share it. (17)*

It was suggested that one way to ensure understanding and recognition of the needs of women workers would be to educate employers.

> *I think that actually it would be very useful if middle managers and supervisors could spend time in aged care, just do visits for example, really see what a carer's life is like, both paid and unpaid care. Employers are always better at this when they have a direct experience and so are educated about the reality of women's lives in particular. (16)*

Flexible working conditions

Having established the principle that workplaces should be environments where workers could expect an understanding of their caring commitments and where there was an acceptance of the legitimacy of fulfilling one's family responsibilities, participants passed on to recommendations for practical changes that would support the carer in specific and tangible ways. The most important was flexibility. The opportunity to negotiate flexible working hours was seen as an important provision, that would alleviate many of the difficulties the women were facing.

> *More flexible working hours which reflect the reality of women's lives and their care responsibilities. Work is still constructed around a male nine to five worker with a wife at home. Most families don't operate like that. People don't have care needs which are pre eight am and post six pm. My mother-in-law's needs were from eight to eleven and then from three to five. Which is precisely when I wasn't around, and we couldn't get services to come at those times. (16)*

> *Recognising that not everything needs to always be done between nine and five. So, although I don't need to do that because of the flexi-time situation here, there are things that I could be doing out of hours to give me time during the day to go and do something else. Client contact needs to be done during reasonable hours, but there's a lot of admin. stuff that doesn't need to be done between nine and five. So to have that flexibility would be really helpful. (29)*

The point was made on a number of occasions that in most cases it would not be all the time that flexibility was needed. However, having the option to work in a flexible way during times of stress and crisis was important.

> *People have the right to work and even just a bit of flexibility and understanding... I mean it's not going to happen every day of the week that you suddenly get called on for something. But if there's enough flexibility, I think if we can do it here, where we've got a place that has to be manned twenty four hours a day, seven days a week and we cope quite well just being flexible when there's a need. I think any employer can do it and with that little bit of support... (27)*

When crises and emergencies arise, workers need to be able to take time off.

> *Realising that carers are under a lot of stress for a start and I suppose just being supportive and allowing time off if necessary, if there's a crisis and really allowing the person to have time off. (30)*

In addition, understanding by employers, that if the work was to be done, it could only be done efficiently if the problems that had arisen at home were sorted out.

> *I guess the way my present employer is, understanding, and realising that they do need to perhaps let me go at the drop of a hat because if I don't I'm in a mess and they are not going to get any productive work out of me. Let me get it sorted out and once it's sorted out then I can come back. So, again, we come back to the flexible hours. If I do take time off, I make sure I put the extra hours in. Understanding and cooperation. (37)*

The importance of being able to take the time required to fulfil family responsibilities without feeling this would be used against you, or worse still result in the loss of a job was emphasised.

> *I think definitely you have to have support so that you can feel comfortable and happy and so that if anything goes wrong they won't be antagonistic toward you about it. (14)*

Leave provisions

Most of the women suggested introducing carers' leave. This would enable the women to feel they had a right to ask for this leave. At present most of the women utilised their own sick leave to enable them to take time off to care for elderly relatives

Official carers' leave would legitimise the leave taken to fulfil one's family responsibilities and would represent an acknowledgment on the part of the employer that workers have family responsibilities and to fulfil these responsibilities may need to take leave from time to time.

> *I would say that carers' leave is really essential. I needed carers' leave desperately during the stage when my mother-in-law was having her first stroke. Carers' leave would have made all the difference to me rather than doing what I did which was, when she was asleep, hopping onto the word processor, moving my office down to her flat, sitting by her bedside marking essays and so on. That was crazy. Carers' leave would have really made a difference. (16)*

> *Carers' leave. Knowing if I go there and ask her as a favour, I have to think about it ten times before I do it and feel bad enough to have to say it. I feel*

I would get the support, but it's a favour. If they did, it would be a lot easier for me to take my mother to the doctor. (41)

Some argued for extending the definition of sick leave.

Perhaps there may be an extension of sick leave to encompass the care of relatives, if it's an emergency and there is nobody else available. I guess leave without pay. Individual organisations make up their own mind about the possibility of being able to do this for periods of time so that people who need a month or a couple of months away from work may feel that their job is still there. If they can see that crisis period is going to subside and they'd have the security of knowing the job was there. (1)

The option to vary work patterns

Other options suggested were the possibilities for movement between full-time and part-time work (and back again), job sharing, taking leave without pay with the possibility of moving onto the Carers' Pension for the intensive periods of caring and utilising long service leave provisions before one was, strictly speaking, eligible to do so.

If there's more part-time work available to people I think this would help and I think it is already happening. Part-time work ***has*** *become much more possible for many people. At certain stages of life that might be more feasible, more appropriate. It depends on a whole range of individual circumstances. Probably we're heading more in that direction. More people are looking at part-time work by the time they are in their forties and fifties and are caring for elderly relatives. (1)*

Some of the women suggested the possibility of job sharing as an option that would suit those with caring responsibilities.

Flexibility. There's not a lot of part-time work out there in the community because here in Australia bosses haven't realised that there are a heck a lot of people who would prefer to work permanent part-time, or to share a job. We have very few people who are prepared to let people share jobs. It would suit a lot of people, solve a lot of unemployment. To have the flexibility of a shared job would be great and employers would actually get six days worth of work instead of five because I've done it, nobody can work six days a week

> *for any great length of time without their health suffering in one way or another. (12)*

The opportunity to take leave without pay for periods of time was another option.

> *I think leave without pay. People being aware that in a CV (curriculum vitae) there may be this great gap which isn't looking after children, which is regarded as okay, is okay. (36)*

As well the possibility of early access to long service leave should be considered.

> *In my case as a long term employee I've had access to things like long service leave. I suppose one possibility would be to enable people to take in a sense before they have earned it. (39)*

Other suggestions for reforming the workplace

Other suggestions included access to a counsellor in the workplace. This person, it was suggested, could well act as a go-between, mediating between the employee and her manager.

> *A staff counsellor where you could go and talk. You don't want to burden your friends with this sort of thing. A staff counsellor would be a wonderful help for any one of us with any problems to have to talk to. One of the things I found very hard, especially in the initial stages was going and telling people and not bursting into tears. I know they don't mind if I burst into tears, but I minded. I know we are talking about only one workplace level and you are looking at a whole variety, but students can go to the counsellor and they'll send many letters stating the reasons that this student should have an extension of time. Perhaps that could help. (36)*

Some women suggested that the provision of workplace based stress management courses would assist them to cope with the day to day stresses and emotional strain of juggling work and family responsibilities.

> *Maybe organised relaxation courses would be a big help. (37)*

Having little training sessions in relaxation and positive thinking and self-esteem, coping with this, that and the other; just help build up that whole person rather than just give them a job. I think if a person begins to feel supported and worthwhile it just gives them more capacity to cope with what comes day by day. (27)

Providing the opportunity for women working and caring to talk with others in the same position, encouraging networking and possibly starting a support group in the workplace for those working and caring, were also mentioned.

Really important would be a support group for people who work. A support group where you can get together and talk about the ups, the downs and the common problems; be able to share experiences and knowledge. It doesn't have to be an organisation. It just needs to be there for people to get that moral support from each other. In the community that is missing for carers. That it is a very big thing. (12)

Some of the women needed somewhere quiet and private to go during the day, so they could rest and recuperate after disturbed nights. At present these women retreated to their cars for some privacy and space during their lunch hour.

Sometimes I've just been through so much and in my lunch time I would like to be able to go somewhere and have a little lay down, somewhere private, and have an hour's sleep. I know there's one girl here that goes and lays in the car and does that, but I couldn't do that. I feel there should be a little area. (7)

Access to a telephone, with privacy, is important.

What I would like is better access to a 'phone so that if you do have to make a private phone, call you don't have to bend over backwards to ask people. For instance, the other day I had to say I have the surgeon ringing me, you must bring me to the phone, rather than being given a message. They're not very diligent in doing that. I think everybody deserves the right of having a phone should they need it and to be able to speak in privacy. (22)

I'm sure all workplaces say, "No personal phone calls", but that's rubbish. We all do, especially staff people. I mean, I have to be in contact with my mother to make sure when she is at home, she's okay. I have to be accessible if she needs me. (17)

Skills acquired as a carer and their relevance to performance at work

This research had assumed the need for one very particular change in workplaces; recognition of skills acquired informally. Skills acquired through education, formal qualifications, training and experience on the job, are generally recognised and rewarded in the workplace. Skills acquired through informal means, "life experience", volunteer work, childcare and child rearing, caring for the elderly or the disabled, are not universally seen as relevant to paid work and are not readily recognised or rewarded.

It is not just that employers have failed to acknowledge the special skills and aptitudes associated with the domestic realm, it is clear that women, themselves, typically have some difficulty in seeing what they do as skilled or in any way special or out of the ordinary. As other research has demonstrated, actually naming and recognising the skills women possess as a result of their domestic, child care and other family responsibilities has not come readily. "Women have proved particularly reticent in acknowledging their unpaid caring activities, let alone claiming for them" (Cox & Leonard 1991, p.16).

One of the participant's illustrated this clearly and played down her skills describing them as...

> *Nothing out of the ordinary... (18)*

She then went on to describe at some length an extraordinary range of skills she had acquired as a consequence of caring for her mother.

The questions asked were, "What are the skills you have developed as a result of your caring activity, that may be of assistance in your work? Are these skills transferable and have you actually utilised these skills in your workplace"?

Thirty two participants had detailed responses and some listed the skills acquired at some length. Eight had little to say and one, as mentioned above, significantly down played the skills.

The skills that they described as particularly useful and important included management, negotiation and organisational skills, most particularly management of time. Complementing these skills were skills in negotiating available options, including a detailed knowledge of and an ability to organise and access a range of services and the skills and ability to deal with and elicit appropriate responses from complex bureaucracies.

> *I have developed skills in negotiating health and welfare systems, giving people information about what's available, what's not available, trends, where there is a lack of money in some areas and so on, and the*

accommodation options. Skills in managing five hundred things at once, priority setting. (4)

You don't realise all the management skills, the time management, your organisation abilities. I do all the housework, all the gardening, the shopping, the cooking. Anything physical, I do it. (17)

(I)n terms of the skills...I suppose a little more patience and understanding. I also cared for my mother when she was dying of cancer and just because I simply had to choreograph what was happening with her medically and liaise with the doctors so that was a real learning experience. I just really had to become the foremost person in her life because my father just dropped his bundle... He was totally unable to do anything. He wasn't able to visit her without someone driving him; he would do nothing. It just all stopped for him and I had to be the absolute strength. I had to do absolutely everything. Organise everything, and just to pull from within, as I think so many women do, you literally pull from the guts and you've got to overcome your own emotions and deal with what has to be and then in your quiet moments you have your cries and so on but you just have to keep stepping above that all the time when the need arises so in terms of certain crises I feel that I would cope better having had that experience. (22)

Along with these skills was the development of astute observation and communication skills, including being able to observe and understand particular behaviours, for example reactions to constant pain, and behave appropriately and sensitively as a result.

Top of the list would have to be things like communication skills, to be able to read people, to be able to read between the lines and realise today this person is well enough to start getting tea ready. Just by walking in the door, to be able to assess a situation and realise that they've had a really "shitty" day. They might have had their sister on the line who's driven them absolutely balmy and they've been in so much pain they haven't been able to move and it's not a very good day to come in and say, "hello" bright and chirpy, because all you are going to get is growls, or don't talk to me. Observational skills and picking up the cues and almost psychic skills, if you can put it that way. To me that's on the top of the list. Being a good communicator even to the point of being able to pick up on cues when people are angry, almost like conflict resolution, that kind of thing, you learn a lot of PR. Most people would think you learn how to do all the manual caring things, and sure you learn those, but it's the other things that go along with it. It's the management of money when there's not a lot of money there, the management of budgets, the PR type work and liaison work, where you've got to liaise with the community worker, the doctor, the chemist for that person, without them feeling as though you are taking over. You have to let them speak, but you've also got to be able to set it all up somehow. So, there are skills there that a lot of people don't necessarily have or realise could be there. (12)

Other skills described were the development and recognition of particular qualities in themselves, such as an increase in their levels of understanding, compassion, empathy, patience, tolerance and kindness, the sorts of qualities that we supposedly value in our society, and the sorts of qualities that we know assist in developing and ensuring good working relationships between people.

I hope I'm more tolerant. I hope I'm more patient. I'm not as angry with other people. I get angry with myself, but I don't think I'm as angry with other people and I don't think I get as upset over - certainly not small things - like I used to. I've learned a lot about older people. I've learned a lot more about illnesses. One of the biggest things I've learned is to be non-judgmental which is very hard. (14)

I can understand and empathise I have a tremendous amount of sympathy for what my mother is going through. (17)

In addition to these qualities, some described graphically the ways in which their caring had provided them with first hand insights into the ageing process,

Well, I suppose, I've got quite a good understanding of elderly people and the ageing process. The fact that elderly people are also very frightened of getting old, being left alone and having no one to care for them. (30)

They had also developed a sensitivity to the importance of maintaining the personal autonomy, dignity and independence of elderly people and had found ways of accomplishing this.

I suppose thinking of her wellbeing; thinking of her nutrition; thinking of her hygiene; thinking how to keep mother as comfortable as possible and as independent as possible. And, I suppose, (learning) not to get depressed. (20)

Allied to these insights were very practical skills that they developed, nursing and personal care skills, bathing, dressing, lifting, feeding, podiatry, administration of medication and ensuring the person being cared for felt safe and secure.

> *She gets a lot of physical support... I assist her showering, I assist her generally. She can manage to get herself dressed in the mornings and undressed. (17)*

> *What do I think is the most important? It's caring for her; making sure that mentally she feels safe and secure, that she's clean, that she's fed, she eats well and she's got plenty to read, all those sorts of things. Also, trying to keep her being able to move and not to seize up and all the things that go with that, getting into the shower and drying her and washing her hair. (20)*

> *Physical skills, such as being able to bath someone. (19)*

Those working in the community services sector, Homecare managers and workers, hospital nurses and those working in nursing homes described the ways in which they utilised the skills acquired in their role as carers in their client contact, in dealing with families and relatives of clients, and the understanding they had of the levels of anxiety and emotional strain the relatives were experiencing.

> *It's taught me a lot about independence and it's encouraged me to try and encourage staff in their attitudes to people to not take over their lives. People need to feel they are in control of their lives and if they don't, they may as well toss it in. They have just then become dependent, so what's it all about if you are not in control of your own life? So it's that sort of thing that I've experienced with my parents and I've experienced as I always have with them, great modelling, great modelling about how you can approach what life is doing to you... I'm experiencing for myself what I am asking my carers to do, go out and help people in my mother's situation and it's just more real somehow, it's just not theory any more. (33)*

> *I've been working in aged care for quite a while but it helps to understand my clients having had personal experience of elderly and unwell people in my mother and father. But then, it goes around and comes around; both help each other. I'm sure having personal experience of relatives being ill, hospitalised, even dying gives you some insight into what it's like for my clients. But also having worked in a nursing home I learned things there that*

> *I'm able to transfer onto how I deal with my family So, it works both ways. (29)*

> *I did find that actually, having my father in a nursing home, made me appreciate other people and their families and what they were going through. When I was working in a general hospital, people would come in and be very, very concerned about their family having to go into a nursing home. And I could honestly, because I'd had the experience, tell them what to expect, what they would have to do, that it wasn't going to be the end of the world and their financial situation wouldn't be really badly off, depending on where that person was going to go of course, and that they would cope. I went through the same feelings of putting dad in (a nursing home) that I'd deserted him. You could reassure people that they would go through those feelings but really in the long run that the elderly person would be better off. (40)*

> *I think because of my particular job I can understand other people in this position. I can understand the tiredness; I can understand the frustration; I can understand that you get angry and you lash out not because you don't love the person, but because of the circumstances. I can understand that. (25)*

In addition to caring for parents, some of the carers also had to deal with dramatic and painful changes in the relationship. In some instances the parent had become very dependent on his or her daughter. It requires considerable skill and maturity to deal with changes of this nature.

> *I've learned how to handle her. You grow up and your Mother is someone you respect but you never see her naked; you never bath her especially in the most intimate part. You never do that. When it happens and you've got to do it, it's not pleasant the first time. To me, she's my baby. I put her in the shower and I bath her as if she was my child. I couldn't do that in the beginning. I've learned how to handle her as if she's my daughter. I undress her; I put her in the shower; I wash her; I dry her; I dress her just as if she's my daughter and I think of her as a dependent. Now I find, because I've got this knowledge, I can do it out there no problem. I've learned how they behave. I know how her mind works. I've learned how an Alzheimer brain works. I've learned the things that she likes, the things that she's unhappy with. She doesn't like being touched, so we avoid touching her, even the kids... Those skills that are acquired are like mother to daughter relationship in reverse. And we make her walk even if she doesn't want to. We just take her for a walk around the house and that keeps her legs moving. Other skills? Maybe how to feed her, which is a totally different. You have to mash*

things. And you've got to always be on the lookout where she is, like a child. (11)

They also developed detailed and useful knowledge about particular illnesses and conditions as well as the ability, skills and confidence to care for those suffering from a range of conditions, for example, Alzheimer's disease and other forms of dementia.

*I've had to change some of my social skills. I recognise that because my relationship with my mother was always a talking one, when she comes down - she'll pop in twenty to thirty times during the day if I'm here - I used to feel like I had to have a conversation with her and with someone with Alzheimers that's extraordinarily difficult. I've now reached the stage I'm quite happy to have her come into the house and I then proceed to just continue on around her with what I'm doing and she has a little sleep. That's been quite a challenge for me, to change my approach. I don't know whether that's a skill, but to change other verbal skills. I find it terribly difficult to say things that aren't true, but sometimes with her it is much easier to agree to an untruth, to say things that aren't completely true. I don't tell her if we are going to be away, because she'll be rattled. Now I have found that a very difficult adjustment to make and I was not good at it for quite a while and I would say things which would then upset her. So, those listening skills because I recognise that (with) a lot of the things that she says, I've got to listen to what she's really trying to say underneath. So, I now recognise that when she comes down and says to us, "You've got the house on the market, when are you going, how do I look after the animals while you are away?", which she would do time and time again, constantly there's that theme, now that theme means, "I'm afraid you are going to leave me". Now I've heard that underneath so all I say to her is, "Don't worry we won't leave you, you are fine, you are safe". She hears that, so I guess those listening skills, listening to what is **really** being said and that's not always easy to find out... I think I've always had that skill but it's been refined, in a sense, because you are listening to this terribly confused, sad message that's coming through. She will ask me about her son - my brother died when he was fifteen, thirty five years ago - and I couldn't understand what she was saying to me and I'd explain logically all about that and then she said to me only a few weeks ago, I know all of that, but (R...) always seems so young". I thought, how stupid of me! Her memory obviously is when he was fifteen. I couldn't hear what she was saying, but I knew that I wasn't giving the right answer; so those skills have improved. I guess too probably a skill in compartmentalising my life. And I've always been a fairly emotional person, I find that I cry even more easily than I ever have and I'm not concerned about that. I can get quite*

> *teary in all sorts of situations and I can handle that. So, I guess, those empathetic skills, that empathising with people, has increased. (21)*

> *I think that really the most important skills are knowing how to handle this dementia problem, not being patronising, keeping their self respect, not demeaning them, just trying to tread that fine line between directing them and understanding. Knowing and understanding what is happening, how to handle it. (13)*

And dealing with specific conditions and illnesses, such as strokes, diabetes.

> *Well, I've learned how to handle stroke patients. I had to. And I can understand how people get angry with the hospital system. I can understand how people get angry with doctors. (25)*

> *I picked up a good basis of medical knowledge. She's diabetic. It's all the associated things that come through long term use of the drugs. (17)*

And with blindness.

> *Caring for the blind, which is not what you are taught as a RN (i.e., registered nurse). You don't have any blind skills whatsoever. You are just told that a blind person is not an abnormal person in nursing, that they are human beings with feelings and sensitivities. But you don't get any actual care of the blind, how to walk with them, how to approach them, how to feed them, how to instruct them where objects are. You get no training whatsoever. I attended the blind society. They had an open day and I spoke to the public relations officer and they just taught me the simple skills of dealing, how you approach a blind person, how you announce yourself, opening a door, where you stand, how they guide. I found that definitely adds to this job, particularly with debilitated people as a result of injury. You just find that you use your blind skills. (10)*

Many also acquired a detailed knowledge of medical terminology, drugs and pharmacology and skills and experience in administering medicines. Some had engaged in careful research on particular medications to ensure they were suitable.

> *I increased my knowledge in pharmacology, in knowledge of drugs and interaction, but mainly because it always interested me. The girls I work with*

will automatically turn to me as a book of knowledge rather than look it up. Mum was on twenty six medications a day. So, I increased that knowledge which I found advantageous when I came here. (10)

Medical terminology, the things I learned from my Dad's heart and lung condition and from Mum's osteoporosis and because I work in a medical field that's probably been a bit beneficial there as well. I can check terms and if I want to know something about a medication I go to the MIMS and look the thing up. (12)

They transferred skills learnt in dealing with crises that arose in their caring role to their place of work. They felt able to deal competently with people confronting similar situations in the paid work environment.

I've learned that I am able to cope. I can't afford to panic when there is a lot of work, because I'm used to knowing what my priorities are and having to deal with that. And if there are any upsets, (being) able to take it in and then let it out later on but know that you have to be (firm). So, in a way you really do toughen up. (41)

Many of the skills spelt out by our participants are of particular relevance to community services and the health sector in which a large proportion were employed. These skills were, in general, the first to be mentioned. They related to personal characteristics and the development of understanding and self knowledge. Thus qualities such as sensitivity, patience, tolerance and compassion were stressed. But there were also those more particular insights such as a greater understanding of the ageing process, the ability to empathise with others and skills in maintaining, as far as possible, the personal dignity and autonomy of the person being cared for. Practical skills were also emphasised. These can be just as "taken-for-granted" as those general "caring" qualities. The specific skills required in providing personal care, in bathing, dressing and feeding those unable to manage these tasks themselves and the development of quite detailed knowledge of particular conditions and skilful administration of appropriate treatment, these were listed as well.

Others are skills which might be seen as being of more general relevance in employment settings beyond the human services sector. In this category one might place practical skills in negotiation and management both of people and of time, skills in dealing with complex and stressful situations. The enhanced observation and communication skills noted by our participants are also qualities that are perceived more generally as contributing to efficient and productive work environments.

What we are arguing is that both groups of skills are of more general value, that they would enhance the development and maintenance of good working relationships in any workplace. While it was the "people skills" that our participants tied quite explicitly to the type of paid work they were doing and while it was these more caring capacities and competencies that they were able to see as transferable to their particular areas of employment, we would want to underline the need for such insights and skills in all areas of work. All work environments gain from the valuing and incorporation of skills and knowledge of the kind that these women were able to offer largely as result of their unpaid caring work and of their attempts to juggle the competing demands of their lives. Workers with such skills are valuable workers.

Conclusion

An analysis of the accounts of paid work and its place in the lives of our participants reveals a number of significant points. All the accounts emphasise the importance of work. Almost all reveal decisions concerning choice of work, promotion and further education and training which have had a detrimental impact on current earning capacity and on possible retirement income. No workplace described in these accounts gives formal recognition to the obligation to care for frail elderly relatives and none has developed explicit policies to address this issue. While a number of workplaces were supportive, the provisions that allow workers to respond to the demands of their caring responsibilities were informal arrangements and understandings, dependent on a thoughtful supervisor or supportive colleagues. Some workplaces were simply unaware, oblivious of the domestic situations and caring responsibilities of their workers. A few work environments were positively hostile. Suggestions for improving the workplace and more generally improving the lot of working carers, were very modest.

It is important to reiterate how crucial paid employment was for the majority of women in this study. Work was important for the financial security it provided immediately and in the longer term, into retirement and their own old age. It was also important for the personal satisfaction and identity that it offered. But like the majority of women in paid employment and, indeed, a great many male workers, these women were vulnerable. Their vulnerability was reflected in a number of ways. Those working in the community sector were very aware of the threat to jobs resulting from reduced funding and the requirement that an increasing percentage of income be acquired from private sources. In addition, many were employed in casual, contract and part-time positions. Few were in jobs with high salaries. On the contrary, most of our participants were either in poorly paid jobs or in professions - nursing and teaching - where the higher salaries are only for the "high fliers" or those able to take on more senior positions. If, in addition, you have a major responsibility of care for an elderly relative or relatives, you are likely to be regarded as a less than ideal worker and, in one or two of the situations recounted here, to be vulnerable to dismissal. For all these reasons hanging onto your job can be difficult and, of course, stressful. A few felt themselves to be hanging on by the skin of their teeth.

Managing the array of demands in your day-by-day life is also stressful. It is not only that there are a great many different tasks to accomplish as described in earlier chapters, it is the need for careful judgement, for the constant re-ordering of priorities, for responding to crises or to the ordinary unpredictable things that may happen to yourself and the others for whom you have a responsibility, it is these requirements that drain you. The more people you are responsible for and the more vulnerable those dependents, the more potential for things to go wrong and the more complex the task of re-scheduling your own life. The lives of workers who care are inevitably very full, complex and busy lives.

All those in this study described the careful allocation of time, the prioritising which was essential if they were to continue to work and care. Their private lives were, in general, characterised by more difficult, fraught and arduous challenges than their work lives. Caring work was physically and emotionally more draining and very often required more developed organisational and management skills than the world of paid work. For many of the women the demands and requirements of the workplace were relatively straightforward, quantifiable and easy to handle in comparison with the complex, unpredictable and, occasionally, chaotic demands placed on them as carers.

Most of the women had given a lot of thought to the relationship between their paid and unpaid work, and considered many ways of dealing with the contradictions and difficulties they confronted. As outlined above, the first possibility that was sacrificed was the option to pursue further study or training opportunities or upgrade qualifications. Some of the women refused transfers and had had to ignore opportunities for promotion. Others opted to accept a drop in salary or a job with more flexibility that better meshed with their caring responsibilities. This would reinforce the argument put forward by Bryson (Grieve and Burns 1994, p. 89) that women are prepared not just to accept, but in some instances negotiate, less responsible jobs to accommodate their family responsibilities. Some had sought employment in an area where they would be closer to home or to their parent's home or in which there would be greater flexibility.

The women downplayed the consequences of their decisions in relation to their careers and were philosophical about the future. As those who had children argued, caring for young children had been a stage in their lives when they had to make choices and compromises in regard to work and family responsibilities. The same applied to this stage of their lives and now it was caring for elderly relatives that was a priority. For the present these responsibilities were uppermost, careers could be resumed later.

The likely consequences in the long term of the choices the women have made, are not clear. Some research has been done on the "costs" of career breaks for childcare. We can speculate that similar disadvantages will accrue for these women who have made similar "choices" in regard to care of elderly relatives. We need more specific research to determine the long term effects of these "choices". It is clear, nevertheless, that even those carers who remain in the workforce may incur significant costs which have not been properly acknowledged. Dropping out of paid work is costly; staying in employment but foregoing salary increases or promotion and restricting one's career choices, is also costly. In the final chapter of this report we emphasise the need for a reassessment of our notions of independence and for greater honesty about the costs for carers.

There is also a need for more research within the workplace itself, research which examines how work might be organised to more adequately take account of workers' family responsibilities and how workplace cultures might be transformed so as to accord recognition and legitimation to those family obligations. We have made a start here. The women in this research had their own views about workplace reform. They utilised their first hand experiences, both positive and negative, to draw up a reform agenda.

Overwhelmingly, the women were seeking recognition and understanding, recognition that what they were doing in taking responsibility for the care of elderly relatives was important and understanding that their lives were complex and they had legitimate reason to request some concessions. They wanted to be trusted and supported. It was clear that when this occurred the difference it made was immense. A sensitive and understanding boss was able to eliminate or, at least, reduce much of the immediate stress experienced in less sympathetic workplaces.

It was also clear from the interviews that some of the women in the sample had managed to keep on working only because of support of this kind. Others who were less fortunate had held onto their jobs in spite of rather than because of the attitudes of their superiors.

If there was a basic understanding and acknowledgment that the women's caring responsibilities were legitimate, other initiatives were possible. The suggestions relating to the improvement of conditions included more flexible working hours, part-time work and job sharing, early access to long service leave, having a category of leave, carer's leave, incorporated into awards.

A short list of additional facilities or supports that employers could provide included access to a counsellor, a workplace based support group and improved physical amenities, including somewhere quiet and private to retreat to and, a very important suggestion for some, access to a telephone.

The women were committed and conscientious workers. They were also committed to caring for their families. They wanted to fulfil their responsibility to their employers, their clients or students, on the one hand, and their families, on the other. Both parts of their lives were important to them. The dilemma was how best to combine them, how to sustain both, but also to keep them separate as discussed earlier in the report. The strain involved was greater at some times than at others, for example, when a crisis arose in the circumstances of the elderly parent. But for all the carers in the group, keeping going and ensuring that quality care was provided, while work obligations were also met, was difficult and stressful. The fact that workplaces were, by and large, less than sympathetic to their circumstances increased the stress. Rather than recognising the particular skills they brought from their caring work to their paid employment, their caring obligations were seen as a problem even a liability.

In the final chapter we explore some of the ways our thinking about such notions as "the ideal worker", "independence" and "time wasters", need to change if we are to create more family friendly work environments and if we are to ensure that employers learn to recognise, value and use the skills and talents of workers who care.

9 Community Services

What impact did the provision of community services have on the lives of working women carers?

As has been documented earlier in this study, the objective of this research was not to examine in detail the provision of community services or the adequacy of that provision. Our primary focus was on the way our participants perceived the relationships between their work and family responsibilities, the interface between work and caring, and the ways in which the women negotiated the allocation of time and energy to the various, demanding and competing areas of their lives. It has also been concerned with how they have dealt with the stress inherent in this kind of "juggling act".

However, it is also clear that service provision and government policy have an impact on these relationships and so also on the capacity to cope day-by-day. We incorporated questions on the ways in which the women and their elderly relatives had utilised community services, how they had found out about them and what had been their experience of particular services. We hoped to gain some understanding of the ways in which the nature and quality of the services available in the community had impacted on the lives of the women and their elderly relatives. In this chapter we provide an account of the experience of forty women attempting to obtain support in providing care for their elderly relatives.

From the beginning it became clear that the factor that made the critical difference in access to and choice of support services, was the living arrangements of the carer and her elderly relatives. The wide definition of a "major caring responsibility" employed in this study has meant that our sample included both those whose dependants were co-resident or living next door and those who were not, i.e., where the elderly relative lived some distance away in their own home or in a hostel or in a nursing home.

The living arrangements were as follows. Fourteen carers had relatives in retirement villages, hostels or nursing homes; twelve carers had elderly relatives living with them and thirteen carers had responsibility for elderly relatives who continued to live in their own homes. Among the latter group were two instances where the elderly relative lived next door to the carer. In one further case the mother lived with two of her daughters, moving between their houses.

In relation to service provision. the women who were the most dramatically affected were those carers who lived in the same house as their elderly relatives. As outlined below some of these women discovered that, as they were working, they were not eligible for most support services.

For many of the women a source of considerable anxiety and distress was the refusal of their elderly relative to accept any support services. This became particularly problematic when the carer felt strongly that the elderly person was in desperate need of support services, indeed was jeopardising health and personal safety through his or her refusal.

Some of the women described how they had gone through a gradual process of persuading the elderly person to accept services, building up trust between the elderly and the service providers, until finally there was some level of acceptance of the support. The ways the women described these situations conveyed the fraught nature of the negotiations that were undertaken. The end result was not always a successful outcome.

Significantly, the services that some of the women had found particularly useful, in terms of their own peace of mind, were those that provided a regular check on and monitored the elderly person or where that was a side benefit of regular contact for some other purpose.

Some of the carers in the sample expressed a reluctance to accept or request any services and felt it was appropriate that they purchase the services that were required.

"There is absolutely nothing for working carers"

As already noted, the group in this study that were the most disadvantaged in terms of the provision of support services were carers who were living in the same house as their elderly relatives.

It is perhaps generally assumed by those providing services that elderly people living on their own should receive community support if they need it, whereas those living with co-resident carers do not need the same level of support or, more accurately, that support is already there to hand. If the carer also has a job, it is, perhaps, assumed that she will be able to pay for any outside services required.

Some agencies had policies that explicitly excluded working women, who were living with their elderly dependants, from access to services. The effect of these policies was to exclude, in some instances, women who were carrying heavy caring loads.

One young woman had been caring for her grandmother for a number of years, had just secured her first job and discovered that this meant she was no longer eligible for support services.

> *Homecare came in at first when I started working, but then they stopped because of a change in policy. They cannot come in and look after a person no matter what their condition, for the reason that another person is there, who is working and they seem to think that you can cope... I'd like the system to change a bit because I was very upset when I got the 'phone call from Homecare and they said to me, "Oh sorry, we can't do any more because you are working". I thought, please spare the little brain cells that I have left in my skull. Maybe it sounds selfish, but I think in a few cases they could be a bit flexible. That upsets me. I think it would also help me with my work environment and everything. I've been really upset over the past few weeks about that, very upset about that, because I thought they'd be a bit more helpful, but they weren't. (15)*

For another woman not having access to services for her mother while she worked meant that, if her mother's health deteriorated, she would have to consider institutional care.

> *(A)s far as community resources go, there's really nothing available for a working person, (for example) as far as Homecare goes. You can't provide twenty four hour care. (You need) respite, for example. Say if my mother had a stroke or something, I'd have to resort to putting her in an institution. Who would look after her while I'm working. And I'm not able to give up work; there's no way I can give up work, financially. There's probably nothing really available as far as community resources go, for working people. (30)*

This woman, who worked for Homecare, had moved into her mother's house. She knew this meant that she would not be eligible for services from Homecare.

> *The fact that I'm working and living in the same home, because I know Homecare's policies as far as that goes, which is, if you're working full-time then you turn to private help. I wouldn't qualify, I don't think. If my mother was living by herself, it's different. Obviously Homecare's resources are limited so I know the story there. Even mowing lawns. The fact that I'm living there, she could have someone mow the lawns for example from Home Care but I wouldn't qualify. (30)*

And, from another carer, a succinct summing up of the situation...

There is absolutely nothing for working carers. (12)

Refusal of the elderly to accept services

Refusal of the elderly relative to accept any of the services available was a major problem for several of the women in the study and they discussed this issue at some length. They were clearly "in a bind". On one hand they saw themselves as responsible for the care of the elderly person, and felt that they knew their relatives well and were in a good position to judge whether or not services were required, yet they had no control over whether or not the services were accepted by the elderly.

In a number of instances, the carer had recognised that her relative was not managing well and required services and support beyond that which the carer could provide. She had organised the appropriate service, only to have the elderly person refuse it.

There appear to be a number of reasons for such behaviour. One explanation that the women we interviewed offered was that their parent was reluctant to admit she or he was not coping and might need some assistance. Another was the desire expressed by the elderly that the carer administer to their needs, not entrust these tasks to "strangers". This caused considerable distress and difficulties for both the carer and those being cared for.

Actually my experience is different from what I've read, in that the services are there and not particularly problematic, but they can't get over the threshold where the old person refuses. (31)

She won't accept any of that. My sister is quite capable of organising services because she works with people like that and she could give her all the care that she needs and make her comfortable and that's where it's frustrating. (41)

No, she won't use them, she just won't. I've tried it. There are so many services. There's the day care service. She won't have anything to do with it. (14)

A not uncommon situation was the refusal of the elderly person to accept any form of respite care, leaving the carer unable to take a break.

Respite care is just not something that she would even consider. You dare not go anywhere. (9)

Another common difficulty was the refusal on the part of the elderly person to accept any assistance with personal care, sometimes insisting the carer do the job. It is, perhaps, understandable that people resist an arrangement that would involve having "strangers" carrying out very personal tasks and seeing one in situations which one finds embarrassing or humiliating, but it did not make the job of caring any easier.

I wanted a community nurse to call in once or twice and wash Dad and shower him. His shower is in a bath and he's got to step in it. He won't have it. (37)

Some of the elderly relatives had gradually withdrawn from social activities, depending solely on the carer for social contact. Attempts by the carer to involve the elderly in social activities were resisted.

There are other services that are available, (for example) the Senior Citizens Centre. She won't have anything to do with pensioners. "Oh those silly old goats down there. Wouldn't dream of mixing in with them". And yet they do have a marvellous time. There's so many activities that they do. She won't mix in there. That would be a good outlet for her. (14)

Another pattern was a series of unsuccessful attempts on the part of the carer to organise community services.

We have used community nurses when she had the fractures; it was a success for a while and then she felt that all the community nurse did was stand there and watch her and she felt embarrassed. It was a success in that I could go to work and know that when she had a shower she wasn't alone, but it wasn't a success in that she was embarrassed. It didn't last long. We've been through numerous people who have come in and cleaned for her a bit. We've had gardeners and she gets sick of them and I end up doing the gardens again and then we get another gardener and something else happens. "They don't do it right. You do it much better than they do", and I end up doing it again. We try different things periodically. I wanted to get her connected up with the continuing care team at the hospital, purely and simply because they said to me that really people should get to know them before they get to the stage of needing it because then they are not a threat. I booked her in and everything else and she said, "I'm not having that". Dug her toes in. So that was that. I even contemplated getting one of the girls to come round and have a cup of tea and a chat on Saturday with us when she rostered on, but when my Mum found out what the ulterior motive was, she was not impressed so she cancelled it. That's one of the problems of having somebody who is very with it. (12)

One woman had some perceptive observations and argued that one possible solution would be for the services to have clearer guidelines concerning intervention. She felt that respecting the rights of elderly people to refuse a service, was perhaps not the best way forward, particularly when it seemed fairly clear that the elderly did require some support.

The changes I would make? I think the constraints on community workers about respecting rights and privacy are too libertarian. It's the actual design of community services that leaves the responsibility for making the hard decisions too fluid. If my father could say look what the wicked state has done to me, it has forced me to do this. It would save his face and not put him in the position of having to admit need and ask for help. So that everybody is "pussy footing" around being too tactful and nobody is breaking through the knot. (31)

The problem is complex. It is not a matter of simply providing appropriate, needed and suitable services and supports. There is a strong belief that accepting services from strangers or the state is somehow not appropriate. As we have argued earlier in this book, the expectation that we (especially women) should provide care for family members is strong; "family" are perceived as the appropriate carers.

For some of the elderly and their carers this refusal of services was clearly jeopardising health and wellbeing. When faced with this dilemma, some of the women had attempted to gradually introduce the service. One of the women related the sequence of events that gradually led to an acceptance of support services on the part of her elderly mother.

Then Homecare started to come in but I needed more than just cleaning her house. That was just an additional sort of thing I had to find time to fit in, to do. I used to wait until she was out of the house and then I'd go in like a fairy and clean the house. We started with the woman from Homecare coming just to do a bit of housework and to just have a chat with her and I said that I particularly wanted them to start to give her a shower but I didn't know how it would happen and within a week it was done and quite easily. So then for a period of time she was being showered three times a week and the house was being cleaned. I was still doing meals and those sorts of things and then, the middle of last year, for the first time, we used respite care so we could get away for a fortnight. (21)

Some negotiated at least a partial, although not very satisfactory, acceptance of services.

I've contracted those two people to help me out with Dad, organised Meals-on-Wheels, Homecare for grass cutting - I used to cut his grass - things of that nature. They come out and do that. And Homecare for shopping on Friday and of course I go over. I take him to the doctor and the doctor now comes down to the house. And that's about it. That's all he would permit. He won't permit Homecare to go into the home and clean. (37)

Importance of community services

The experience of the carers outlined above, contrasts dramatically with the experience of the women whose elderly relatives did accept at least some of the services available.

For the women whose elderly relatives were eligible for services, the support they found the most useful was that which could perform a kind of monitoring role. Having someone visit the elderly, daily in some cases, alleviated the stress on the carers of feeling they constantly needed to check on the person being cared for. The contribution these services made to alleviating the carer's anxiety, the knowledge that someone was checking on the elderly person and making sure they were all right, was invaluable. There was, as well, the more tangible help in those cases where the community nurse was able to visit regularly to administer medication and monitor the physical health of the elderly person.

The services that would make a difference are the ones that turn up every day that monitor. Anyone can monitor. It could be Meals-on-Wheels. It could be Homecare. It could be the parish priest or somebody who is prepared to do it... There are so many "at risk" people out there in the community who have problems. Like in Nan's case she had a stroke. But there are other people with similar sorts of things where they really do need that monitoring. (4)

Reluctance of some carers to seek or accept services

Finally, it was not only the elderly dependants who had difficulty asking for or accepting services. Several of the carers also felt this. They argued that having taken on the responsibility to care for their elderly relative they were obliged to manage the care themselves. They didn't feel it was appropriate to seek or utilise community support or services at this stage.

> *I don't think either one of us has reached a stage where we need outside help. I'm aware of all the services that are available but I also feel that I've got obligations as far as my mother goes anyway and even if the community services could give help to working people, I really couldn't see myself resorting to community help at all. (30)*

> *I have an attitude that I have a career and my brother is a professional and my husband is a professional and so far as we've maintained that we feel it's our responsibility not to tap into resources while ever there are people who don't have family to care for them. (33)*

A number could afford to pay for services and felt they should pay. One participant made the point that, through their contribution as carers, they were saving the government money. She had been reluctant to ask for help initially, even though she had realised that some assistance was needed.

> *There was the initial difficulty within myself of overcoming pride or whatever, saying that I needed other people to come in. Having done that I found them very helpful and easy to approach and very supportive. So I have certainly no complaints and a real sense that they were there to be helpful and that they weren't being suspicious that you were trying to rort the system... We were happy to pay for whatever was necessary. Mum's got very good superannuation. There is recognition that there is a responsibility within the community to care, but we also have a responsibility to pay whatever we can afford to pay in that situation. It's helping the community by keeping her in her home rather than the great expense to the community of keeping her in a hospital. In the sense we are doing the health system a service by keeping her in the community for that additional length of time. (21)*

Conclusion

The wide ranging definition of a major caring responsibility which we adopted in this research has enabled us to highlight the very different access to services of co-resident carers and their dependent relatives compared with those carers whose elderly relatives lived in their own homes, hostels or nursing homes. The individuals who "fell through the net" were the working co-resident carers. If the elderly were living in their own homes they were generally eligible for community services, but if they were living with their carers, the carer's status as "employed" excluded both carer and "caree" from access to some support services.

In this instance it would appear that a wider definition of "need" should be employed. For instance, to provide services to one elderly person living in her own home, with a working carer living separately, and to exclude another from access to services on the basis that she lives with her carer, a working women, seems grossly unfair.

The reluctance or refusal on the part of the elderly to utilise support services, presents us with a real dilemma. How should we deal with people who need support services to maintain their health and wellbeing, yet refuse to accept these services? After all, most of us have been imbued throughout our lives with an ethic that places value on independence and self reliance, and would have sympathy with a refusal to have strangers undertaking intimate and personal tasks. On the other hand, what do we do when this refusal means a carer is shouldering unreasonable burdens or, indeed, if the health or safety of the elderly person is compromised? There may even be a case to be made, as one of the participants stated, for compelling some people to accept at least some level of intervention and monitoring of their health and wellbeing to ensure that personal safety and health are not compromised even if by so doing the person's independence is undermined. In this context, questions of rights, of whose rights should be respected, are not easily answered. The rights of carer and "caree" are not always the same and may, in fact, be antithetical.

This dilemma and resulting problems, gives heightened significance to the responses of the carers who found the most useful services were those that monitored the health and wellbeing of the elderly relative. Knowing that someone was visiting the elderly and ensuring they were all right, contributed markedly to the carer's peace of mind.

As the provision of good quality childcare has come to be accepted as being crucially important in enabling the fuller participation of women in public life, so good quality support services for the aged in our society are also critical. Wide ranging services that are well run, well coordinated and well funded are vital both to the elderly in our society who need this support and to those who care for them. They are the mark of a society that truly values the caring work of its citizens, male and female. Such provision is also of importance to those who do not yet and who may never have call upon these services. For all of us they represent a security, a protection, an important counter to that anxiety about our own and our parent's future that is felt, in some measure, by everyone.

10 Conclusion

Like most research that examines complex areas of human experience, this research is really several studies. At one level this is an account of the busy lives of forty women, of their attempts to order those lives, to make sense of them to themselves and explain them to others. At another level it is a practical compendium on coping with the care of an elderly relative; there is here something of a survival manual and a reassurance that others have experienced the same things and often responded in the same way. It is also a study of the day-by-day minutiae of caring and of the satisfaction of caring and the toll that it exacts. It is a study of workplaces and the response from different employers and managers to the caring responsibilities of their staff. It is a reflection on "time" and "choice", on the nature of caring and of stress and on the ideologies that permeate the world of work. It is all of these things. But overwhelmingly it is an argument about how as a society we should respond to the fact that all individuals for some periods of their life will be dependent: it is a significant element of the human condition. Part of that argument, a major part, is about how we support those who take on a major responsibility of care whether for a short time or whether for "the long haul". We have examined only one area of care and by one particular group but the argument is a general one even while it must take account of the diversity within the population of carers.

So this is social policy research rather than an ethnographic study even though it has elements of the later approach. It is concerned with how we go about creating the "good" society and so it must also be concerned with what "good" means. The assumption underpinning this research is that caring is not a peripheral activity for which only some have a responsibility. On the contrary, it is pivotal not only in analytical terms (Graham 1983) but because the capacity to respond to another who is dependent and has some claim upon us is critical in achieving the "good" society. Social policy research, in this sense, is always a moral discourse as well as a more practical exploration of ways of understanding an issue and of attempting to respond to it.

Let us first draw together some of the findings and conclusions of this study. We began with the experience of caring for that was where our participants wanted to begin the account of their lives or at least where they placed the greater emphasis in their stories. This research demonstrates very clearly that while both caring and paid work were of central importance to these women, the significance of relationships in their lives and the strong sense of responsibility they felt for the wellbeing of those who had some claim on their attention, these family issues, shaped their day-by-day existence and the priorities they established in every other part of their lives.

In this sense it might be concluded that there must have been a clear cut decision to take on caring responsibilities and that we could thus pinpoint the moment when the choice to care was made. In general, however, this is not the case. The choice to take on a major responsibility of care was rarely a single and never a simple choice. Choice is almost always circumscribed by factors and circumstances that limit choice. Some of these limiting factors are bound up with notions of what a parent would expect or prefer, or with undertakings given to one parent concerning the care of the other. Sometimes the choice has been determined by the carer's own conviction that it would not be right to place a parent in a nursing home or only if there really was no alternative. If and when they are compelled to take up the nursing home option, care giving continues; it remains a central feature of their lives and continues to frame the other choices they feel able to make.

Choice is constrained by the real options available for the care of an elderly person who has become increasingly dependent. A carer attempting to assess the range of possible caring arrangements may well find themselves concluding that there really is no alternative but to have a parent live with them.

As well, each caring situation has it own history; in some cases a long history. It becomes difficult to establish the one point at which caring was begun. A major responsibility of care has been preceded by times of less demanding care giving. Very frequently these earlier periods are comprised of actions and ongoing support which contribute to the well being of a parent or other elderly relative but which are not necessarily seen as caring activity at all. The majority of the women in this study did not see the choice to care as a single event and a few did not define even their present activity as "being a carer".

Caring in this research, as in other studies, is shown to be a complex activity. It involves "caring about" as well "caring for". The emotional work which the concept of "caring about" attempts to capture, exacts a heavy toll. Both aspects of the caring role contribute to the stress of caring. In this study we document again the array of demands placed upon the carer and demonstrate how frequently carers strive to meet those demands without much help from others. This is so of both formal and informal support networks. In fact "networks" does not describe what most confronted when seeking help in whatever form. As workers they have been, by and large, assigned a lower priority in the provision of community services or, indeed, deemed ineligible for many services. Finding out about what was available and for which services they might be eligible, proved a difficult task even when they were working in the community services sector. In seeking family support they confronted what others have discovered - that most family members do not want to contribute except in relatively marginal ways. Some siblings do not see it as their role to do anything. And among this group of carers were quite a number who were the only "family", in any event.

Caring is stressful work. It is often costly in terms of the impact on the health and wellbeing of the carer. For some that cost is continuous and on going. For others it is associated with particular points of crisis in a history of caring. In either case, when the impact on health has been great, the effects are likely to be ongoing; they continue beyond the crisis and even when the caring itself has come to an end.

These carers were working in paid jobs that may also be stressful in a number of ways. All of the individuals were working in areas that involved a focus on the needs of others. Almost all were working in agencies or areas of the public sector which were under intense funding pressure. Not only did this mean the threat of job loss in a few cases but it was experienced everywhere as the constant pressure "to do more with less". One outcome of this has been that people are working longer and longer hours to ensure the work gets done. While not all of these stressors were experienced by all our participants, there emerges from these accounts a recurring picture of stressful work environments becoming more stressful and difficult as time goes on.

Nevertheless, the world of paid work was depicted as more manageable, orderly and predictable than the world of unpaid caring work. Its demands on time were generally a known factor and life could be planned around that requirement. Caring responsibilities had to be fitted in with the demands of work and most carers spoke of their attempts to keep separate the two spheres of their lives and to try to ensure that they did not let their anxiety about their parent's wellbeing intrude into the work context. None felt they had achieved this separation and, at times, of course, the demands at home or from a frail parent accommodated in a nursing home or hostel, are immediate and pressing. There are crises that require that you drop everything else and respond to that need.

For some the separate nature of the world of paid employment was a welcome relief. There you could immerse yourself and for a time be a person separate from the demands of family; it provided an escape from the stress of caring. Others found the pressure to retain a separation simply added to the stress. They would have welcomed the possibility of a break from work, a reduction in hours at least for a time. But for the majority of our participants dropping out of paid work, even for a short time, was not really a possibility. What is important to underline is that work was important for these women. For some it was immensely important personally and many spoke about how much they enjoyed what they did. For most it was also financially vital that they continue to work and to work full-time.

These women faced a fundamental dilemma. They wanted to be able to provide a reasonable quality of life for their parents or grandparents for as long as it was possible for them to do so. They wanted, also, to continue to work, for their immediate and long term security and for personal satisfaction. Sustaining both these areas - of work, and of response to another's need - was difficult to achieve at particular times in their present lives and for most there was a fear that there may come a time when it would not be possible to continue. All had given considerable thought to the future and what they would do if, and when, the health of their relative deteriorated. For most it was clear that dropping out of the paid workforce was not an option.

What was also clear was that for most there had to be considerable adjustment of careers and choices about paid work as a result of caring responsibilities. While few had cut back on hours, all had accepted restrictions and foregone opportunities. For some this took the form of postponing further education or of not undertaking training that was offered. Others decided not to seek promotion to more demanding jobs or not to take a position because it was too far from where a parent lived and would complicate the business of fitting in caring demands. Remaining in employment might be vital for most but actual careers or any notion of planning a future path in the workforce, took a "back seat". Ambitions were not discussed. The cost for some in foregoing education or promotion was very great and had meant a curtailing of any real chance of long term secure income: for others the costs were of a lesser magnitude but the impact on financial security and personal satisfaction was still clearly evident. For a very few, the caring had come at a time when the worker had already attained a senior position and so the impact on career, and thus also on personal finances and sense of achievement, was marginal.

Workplaces responded to the caring demands in a number of different ways but few could be described as truly supportive. There were no formal workplace policies and nowhere had management instigated a discussion of the issues involved. Where there was some flexibility, it was provided by fellow workers with whom a carer worked most closely. There were a very few exceptions to this general picture of inflexibility and lack of support. These were a small number of local agencies of a larger organisation which had as director someone aware of, and sympathetic to, the workers in this situation. These managers ran their agency in such a way as to take into account the caring loads that some of the workers were carrying and tried wherever possible to make adjustments to work schedules and routines to ease the pressure on these women and give them some flexibility. One church based agency also stood out in this respect. In that case, the manager in the central office had a keen awareness of the caring situations of workers in local agencies and facilities and of the pressure on these workers particularly at a time of crisis either in the paid or unpaid work environment. Such sensitivity was, however, rare. The difference that it made in the lives of the workers lucky enough to be employed in these agencies, was immense.

When asked what needed to change in the workplace to better accommodate caring responsibilities, this group of carers made a number of specific suggestions. All were exceedingly modest. No one expected major adjustments or provisions. Nevertheless there was a call for much greater flexibility in the ways managers organise work and schedule workers and for a recognition that the requirement to vary such arrangements and to make allowance for the pressures on a worker who is caring for an elderly relative, are usually of a minor nature. Where the variation needed is of a major kind, then it is usually necessary only for a short period, to accommodate a temporary crisis. The possibility of working from home for short periods was mentioned by a number of participants. Other provisions included more flexible pensions able to be made available quickly and for short periods of caring when a crisis arises. More and better respite and day care provision was emphasised and more adequate funding of community services in the area of aged care. Formal support services that are dependable, flexible and properly staffed are important to all carers including those who work full time. Without proper support services, it is difficult if not impossible for carers to sustain the caring demand.

The picture that emerges from this study is of a particular group of workers who for the most part are under much greater stress than their co-workers, those who are not, for the moment, carrying a major responsibility of care for an aged relative. The stress is associated with attempting to juggle the demands of paid work and unpaid caring work. This struggle was compounded by the fact that work was often stressful and caring almost always so. In addition, most carers in this study had other demands on their time as well, the most common and important being the care of children. Like most other women they also managed the domestic arrangements at home, tried to keep up with friends and to make a contribution in the community at large. Leisure, hobbies and time to self did not feature prominently in the lives of these women.

What also emerges is a picture of conscientious workers. While the greater emphasis in the accounts was on the caring work and its particular demands, it was equally clear that doing one's job well and being effective and achieving in the paid workforce, was important to these women. They were serious workers wanting to be enabled to do their work and to care well at the same time.

Reflections on caring and work

Looking back over this particular study and reflecting on the accounts of these women we have found ourselves preoccupied with some important recurring issues. Many of these issues we have seen emerge in earlier studies we have undertaken and also, of course, in the research of others. But some themes and ideas seem to be associated more particularly with the circumstances of both working and caring or given more telling expression in this context. So our earlier reflections on the problematic nature of choice and the significance of time in caring take on new meaning. Our understanding of the stress of caring has been enhanced and enlarged. How we conceptualise dependence and independence is revealed even more clearly as needing to be reassessed. How we construct the notion of an ideal worker or ideal manager or model work place must be re-examined. All of these reflections might be judged interesting and important in their own right but our concern here is with how we change work places, government policies and community attitudes so as to create a better and more supportive environment for workers who are caring, and indeed, for all workers and all carers.

So in this, the final section of our book, we want to set out some of the more significant of our reflections on caring and paid work, and juggling the two.

The nature of caring

This study has raised anew concern about the nature of caring and the ways in which caring is conceptualised in our society. There are a myriad of issues here. Let us consider just a few of them.

Caring has been defined in much social policy as referring exclusively to co-resident caring. Along with this notion has been an assumption that it is a full time activity. Our research would call into question so limited a view of caring. Not only were all our participants in the paid work force, many were caring for relatives who were still living in their own homes and quite a number had care of a parent in hostel accommodation or a nursing home. We are not speaking here of a low level of care or of short periods of intensive care after hospitalisation or during an illness. One requirement for inclusion in our research was that the participant be carrying a major and ongoing responsibility of care. Having a relative in a hostel does not mean that you are thereby acquitted of any responsibility for the care of that person and the level of demand in that caring may be considerable and sustained. This is particularly likely to be the case when a parent is concerned rather than a more distant elderly relative.

It is important that we distinguish between a major responsibility of care and, what Lewis and Meredith have called, "semi-care" (1988, p. 181). But this does not mean that the latter is of little consequence. It is also important that in calling for greater recognition in the workplace of that whole range of caring responsibilities associated with the different stages of the life cycle, that we do not ignore or downplay the lesser levels of care or short term caring demands. Both can be, and usually are, stressful experiences; the emotional load can be considerable.

It may well be useful to see carers as falling into one of four categories, and of course they may move between them at different stages in their caring history. These groups could be called major carers, those involved in semi-care, monitoring carers and short term crisis carers. The definitions of these groups will, undoubtedly, be further developed in later research, but the names chosen for the categories give some clue to our thinking here.

* Major carers care for relatives who may need help with bodily necessities like "toileting" and eating. Such a relative may be resident in a nursing home, hostel or co-resident with the carer. The time demand is considerable and constant or, at least, very regular.

* Semi-carers may care for someone who needs help with shopping and heavy cleaning and is perhaps living in an adjacent suburb or in a hostel or in a retirement village.

* Monitoring carers may need to visit the relative every week and telephone more regularly "to keep an eye on things".

* Short term crisis care is self explanatory and is usually associated with recovery after hospitalisation or any serious illness.

We would also emphasise, again, the fact that caring is rarely if ever a straightforward and unproblematic "choice". There is clearly a sense in which individuals "choose" to care and deliberately and willingly take on those responsibilities. But, as already emphasised, it is also the case that quite frequently there are in fact few real choices "out there" and indeed few options in one's own mind. Many people have strong feelings about the obligation to care and some have given undertakings to parents that they will be cared for in their own home, or their child's home, for as long as possible. Some parents refuse to consider any alternative but that of remaining in their own home and not a small number refuse to consider receiving help from the kinds of community services which are designed to enable them to do so. A daughter or son is placed in a very difficult situation in such circumstances. Most would find it difficult if not impossible to stand back and ignore their parent's real and immediate need for care even when the impact on their own lives may be verging on the disastrous. And indeed, deciding just how one is to intervene in such situations, as a daughter or grand-daughter or daughter-in-law, is not at all straightforward.

Re-conceptualising caring means that we accept that caring is rarely marked by any single "choice" and that it reflects and is shaped by an ongoing, close and often complex relationship. Not only is there a history to any caring situation, each is a relationship and each represents a stage in that long history which characterises adult family relationships.

Caring is not one uniform experience; on the contrary it is multi-faceted. Not only does caring comprise a vast range of physical tasks, it entails an emotional involvement that is, in the view of our participants, the more stressful aspect of the caring giving role. As we note at a number of points in this research, this has been described as "caring about" as distinct from "caring for". It means being available, listening to, taking time with the person, being attentive as well as attending to their physical needs. This in an important distinction to make. Caring about someone means that you are never entirely without some anxiety as to their well being. It is not solely a question of the time taken to perform the physical tasks of caring, it is the recognition that to care for someone is to carry with you concern for that person's needs at every moment of the day, including while at work. It is also important to make the point that you may "care about" someone without necessarily being the person who does the "caring for" that person or who performs *all* of the physical work involved in caring for that person.

The separation of work and family care

And this brings us to a second significant and recurring issue in our research - the obligation felt on the part of workers to keep separate the two primary spheres of their lives, paid work and family responsibilities. We have already mentioned that while many of the participants in this study spoke of their attempts to separate out these different areas of obligation, none felt that they had achieved it. That such a compartmentalising of one's life should be seen as desirable, and certainly that is what is posited, is noteworthy and bears further analysis.

We would contend that not only is this compartmentalisation of the significant areas of one's life an impossible and indeed undesirable goal and that for women in the circumstances we were exploring often a very stressful one as well; we would want to press the argument further and argue that it has destructive consequences for all of us.

It is important to emphasise again that there are some contradictory elements here. As we have already observed, for many of the women in this study as for many other women, work has provided an escape from the onerous and restrictive nature of caring work and from the stresses associated with care giving. A number were quite explicit about this and claimed that they would "go mad" if they had to give up work and care full-time. In that sense it was good to be able to throw oneself into one's work and seemingly forget the difficulties, and not infrequently the distress, involved in caring for a parent who was becoming increasingly dependent. But the separation of work and caring is a rather different exercise when it is embraced as a survival strategy. When, however, it is part of a mind set, an organisational culture, that operates in workplaces across the globe and which compels workers to act as though there was no home and family, as though there were no caring responsibilities, then what we are dealing with is a very destructive mythology. We can note here only briefly some of the significant consequences that flow from this construction of our social world.

We have noted already the stress involved in the very attempt to live up to this expectation. This stress is additional to the strains of the caring work itself and the demands of the job.

There is another consequence we want to emphasise and this impacts upon us all and leaves us all the poorer in terms of the work environments we might want to encourage. This is the basis we use to define the "good" worker or the worker who is serious about his or her work. We would suggest that in large measure we have taken for granted that a characteristic of the "good" worker is that he or she is "one hundred percent" dedicated to his or her work and that this dedication is evidenced both in terms of the availability to work when needed and in a lack of domestic distractions, a freedom from the demands that family members may make. Before we consider in more detail just what this characterisation represents, let us note some significant consequences that flow from organisational cultures which are premised on particular and narrow notions of the serious worker and of the obligation to keep separate one's paid employment and unpaid caring work and family responsibilities.

The first is that only men (or those with wives) or women without children or dependent parents can be serious workers; they have minimal family responsibilities. The research we describe here does not address the question of the caring responsibilities of men but it is important to question the assumption that men are freed up to work without any great concern as to the welfare of their children, spouse or parents. After all, men are also members of families with, it must be assumed, a vital interest in their family's wellbeing.

The second assumption is that women's employment can best accommodate their family's needs if they work in a part-time or casual capacity. Those in full-time work are "suspect"; they may take off at any time to have children or to attend to their children's needs and so promotion to management positions and training are unnecessary or not a good investment from the employer's point of view. While clearly there has been some undermining of this ideology in recent years, in Australia as elsewhere, there is also abundant evidence that it remains a powerful mind set. The very lack of women in senior positions in industry, the public service, universities and unions, is, in part, a reflection of this view of "the proper order of things".

Questioning such notions of the proper order of things is particularly important in the current context of these economically troubled times with high rates of unemployment, much uncertainty and market volatility. It is also difficult. We are not able here to explore these significant issues in the detail they deserve. We do, however, make one vital point. Carers in this study spoke of the need for greater flexibility in the workplace so that when there is a crisis or if the caring demand increases, they can legitimately request some adjustment of hours or work load. In some cases such an adjustment might need to be for a lengthy period but in by far the majority of cases, the flexible arrangement is short term, designed to meet a crisis. The concern is that the need for flexibility will only be addressed in terms of permanent part-time work or "casualisation" of positions. For the majority of these workers, this could not be considered an appropriate response to the need for flexibility in the workplace. We will return to the question of flexibility.

The concept of the ideal worker

If, as we are arguing here, there is a need to reassess conventional notions of the necessary separation of work and family and of the appropriate working arrangements for women, then there must also be a fundamental reappraisal of what constitutes the ideal worker. At the same time, it seems fitting that we reconsider what it is that constitutes the ideal "manager". Such reassessments become as well, an argument about efficient and productive workplaces. This has become a critical argument in Australia. What constitutes efficiency and productivity has not been argued with the rigour and care we might wish. It is a debate that social scientists, especially sociologists, must also address more adequately than they have to date.

If we pursue the argument concerning what constitutes the ideal worker then it quickly becomes clear that the stereotype of the ideal or serious worker runs directly counter to the flexible, cooperative and innovative worker described as essential to the modern manager, employer or business unit. It also becomes clear that this argument taken to its logical conclusion brings us, finally, to an absurd position. Stated baldly,

* desirable or ideal workers are workers who do not take a major responsibility for what goes on in the home which they occupy, on average, more than one hundred hours in any week;

* ideal workers are workers who have no detailed knowledge about, and do not have to concern themselves with, the management of the domestic sphere of their lives and what knowledge they do have, is mediated through another, usually a wife;

* ideal workers are not required to have developed any real understanding of, or feeling for, or skills in, dealing with children, sick people, people with a disability or the elderly;

* ideal workers do not, should not have to, care *for* people even if they care *about* them.

To this list might be added another insight that a number of writers have dwelt upon in detail;

* ideal workers are not seen to have need of those skills which particularly

> pertain to the private sphere - nurturing skills, a vicarious capacity, a predisposition to think of the welfare of others and to attend to their needs, altruism, patience, listening skills, encouragement and affirmation of others, "emotional work". These skills are apparently not required to be exercised in the world of work.

This is, of course, nonsense and we all know it to be so. Why then do everyday notions of what is ideal in a worker continue to incorporate so distorted a picture of what is admirable in human beings? Why is this conventional notion of the serious worker so at odds with what the current literature in management sets out as desirable traits and capacities in a manager? To answer these questions would require a study on its own and we cannot even begin to address them here.

The nature of dependency

Let us turn instead to a consideration of the third significant issue - the understanding of dependency. This was also a recurring theme in the research although not quite so explicitly stated by our participants as the other two.

Dependency is a part of the human condition and all are dependent for periods of our lives. Yet, in our society, dependency is viewed as an undesirable and negative state; self sufficiency and independence are venerated. This creates some problems and results in much confused thinking on the subject. In general, there is little difficulty in viewing enforced dependency as undesirable and something that takes from a person's humanity. We do not, however, always see this state for what it is. When many women and, less frequently, men forego paid employment to care for someone who cannot care for themselves, they become themselves dependent. They and, very frequently, the one for whom they care, must rely on someone else for their material support, usually either a partner or the state.

As already emphasised, the women in this study were more than aware of the implications for their long term security and independence of remaining in the workforce. They viewed with very great reluctance the idea of even a temporary retreat from the workforce to care for their elderly relative. For many even temporary unemployment was not an option. They could not have met their financial obligations on a carer's pension. But the long term prospects were even more grim. The likelihood of being able to move back into the workforce when the caring ceased was a remote one. Middle aged workers do not find it easy to re-enter the workforce especially after a break of several years. Poverty in old age was a real possibility for many if they were forced to give up work.

But there is a further dimension to the issue of dependency. Dependency is rarely absolute; independence, never. There are degrees of independence. What became very clear to us in talking to our participants is that many, indeed most, had already foregone "degrees of independence". By this we mean that, as a result of caring responsibilities, the women in this study had sought adjustments in their working lives and had made decisions about promotion and the pursuit of further education or training which have had, and will have, palpable negative effects upon their financial independence. They had made decisions to delay training or further education to upgrade qualifications, they had turned down or not sought promotion, or not taken up the opportunity for new or different work because of the demands of unpaid caring work. In this sense, and we are arguing this is an important reconceptualisation of independence, they have given up a claim upon a higher degree of independence and security both in the immediate future and, perhaps more importantly, in the long term, into their own retirement and old age.

We would add a footnote here concerning the kinds of work in which these women were typically engaged and the sectors of the workforce in which they were employed. A number of the women in our study who were working in the community sector, spoke of their choice to work in a sector that is not characterised by high salaries, job security or assured and predictable career progression. It is also stressful work. There are, however, real attractions to work within this area. The preference for work in the context of small, usually local, organisations which offer some flexibility, work autonomy, flatter structures and small team work, clearly held appeal, although there was no extensive discussion of these concerns in our study.

It is, however, important in a discussion of foregone opportunities for advancement and career progression, to acknowledge that for many women, given the nature of the work they do, these options may not exist or, at least, are likely to be very restricted. Areas of the workforce, such as the community sector, have traditionally been seen to provide little in the way of career structure. We would, however, register a note of caution here. We may well need to re-examine this assumption, an assumption which community workers themselves accept in large measure. There is some evidence that most workers in this sector do have some real options for progression in status, job security and salary. Recent exploratory research by Onyx and Maclean on career progression in the New South Wales community sector, has suggested that we may need to reassess our assumptions about the lack of possibilities for career advancement in this sector (1995, p. 55-70). If they are right, then this adds further weight to our thesis that the cost to workers in terms of a curtailment of their immediate and future independence, is very real and must be recognised. In any event, the choice to work in certain areas of employment, to do "women's work", will usually entail a cost, especially in terms of the salaries these workers are likely to attract.

Time and caring

We have dwelt upon the subject of time and caring at some length in this book. It is hardly surprising. Time and the ways in which it is spent, the sheer lack of time for anything other than the immediate demands of caring and paid work and children and the management of the domestic front, these issues stand out in these accounts.

Time is always an issue in caring. Caring takes time, time to attend to the many different tasks, time just being with the person being cared for, listening time, companionable time. There is never enough time to do all that needs doing. Most especially there is never enough time to do the things that are just for one's self - leisure, hobbies, or simply relaxing. What stands out in this study, however, is that if you work and care, all these factors are likely to be magnified. It is even harder to find time just to be with one's parent and it is just as hard to find time for one's self. Responding to demands that others make, whether at home or at work, is often experienced as all consuming. Paid work, itself, consumes considerable amounts of time and, in the contemporary context, there is an increasing expectation that work can make demands beyond office hours. Caring time operates to a different clock from that of the world of work.

Time is just as fractured and fragmented. It takes real organisational skills to manage the competing demands and to fit into one's life all the different things that need to be attended to, that require time. The unpredictable, the crisis, is even more difficult to contend with, whether the crisis arises in the caring situation or at work.

But what we want to underline at this point in our book, where we are drawing out the main themes in this research and recording our reflections, is that time is a moral issue. Morality is to do with what we value, what we believe is right and good. It is thus concerned with the valuing of some things over other things. Caring raises a number of moral dilemmas for us all. How we spend our time is nearly always judged in moral terms. Devoting time to an activity such as caring is supposedly valued because it requires a degree of altruism and concern for the welfare of others. Caring for one's parent is supposedly a worthy thing to do; it is an important instance of facing up to one's family responsibilities or duties. Not to show any concern for one's parents would be judged by most as immoral, although there is little censure for such behaviour.

But in reality we place little value on caring. It is largely unrecognised and unacknowledged. It is usually assumed that only certain people will be required to undertake this demanding work. Although there are men performing caring roles, it is invariably women who do the bulk of the caring work in our society. It receives no monetary reward. When paid work involves caring, it is invariably less valued than other types of work. If you work and care, it will usually count against you.

To care, and especially to care well, requires time. What elderly people most value is companionable time, time taken to be there with them. Spending time with someone is a way of valuing them, of giving them a sense of being valued. Yet we have given this activity little value and failed to make adequate provision for it in our community services.

There is an additional issue. The fact that some people take up this "moral" duty, the fact that they give up their own time and give it to another, means that all of us benefit. Yet this is rarely acknowledged. The "good society" is one in which people care for one another and supposedly are valued for doing so. Yet our response to the fact of caring has been half hearted and parsimonious. When individuals care for their elderly parents, they save the community considerable sums of money. Carers receive very little in return. The community sector is under-funded. The pension provisions for carers are very meagre indeed. The wages lost by the individual are not seen to be part of the equation. The "degrees of independence" which have been forfeited are never recognised. And, most importantly, the carer, herself, is less likely to viewed as a "good", "ideal" or "model" worker.

Time, productivity and efficiency in the workplace

We make one final comment on the issue of time and this is one that relates specifically to the workplace. We would want to see a more honest assessment of what it is that truly wastes time and creates inefficiencies in workplaces. Each of us could list "favourite" time wasters - unnecessary badly chaired meetings, endless posturing in meetings, ego games and face saving exercises, certain kinds of bureaucratic campaigns in quality management and so-called accountability, over-elaborate performance indicator systems, and so we might go on. There will, doubtless, be some argument among us as to which are the real time-wasters. Our argument is that when a company or agency makes provision for a worker to have time off, legitimately, to take her aged mother to the doctor's or to attend to some crisis that has arisen at home, this is not going to contribute to inefficiency in the world of work or significantly reduce overall productivity. The workers who might avail themselves of such provisions are not less serious workers. There will have to be safeguards against abuse of more flexible provisions in the workplace, but such formal recognition of the legitimacy of the family responsibilities of workers does need to be put in place. It is not the demands of caring or family responsibilities that are unreasonable impositions on employers. These demands reflect the realities of our lives and those that respond to them with diligence and thoughtfulness are workers who should be valued for doing so. There is clear evidence in our research that the employer or manager who recognises, values and supports the caring responsibilities of his or her workers, does not have cause to regret such actions.

Implications for policy and practice

In a concluding chapter to a study of this kind, it has been important to consider what the findings imply for social policy and for professional practice. To consider these implications is to confront two primary areas of concern.

The first relates to the very modest changes in workplace practices and in the delivery of community services which this group of working carers has called for. In relation to workplaces, the plea has been for greater workplace acknowledgment of the nature of family responsibilities, for flexibility in the ways in which work is organised and for specific provisions within the work environment (access to telephones, work based counselling services, quiet rooms, etc.). In the case of community services, the changes that working carers have called for are not so very different from the requests of all carers, for example, for increased provision of respite care, both day care and longer term respite, which is of high quality, accessible, affordable and flexible.

What is of concern is the extent to which changes of this kind, however modest and reasonable, have become more and more unlikely. On the one hand, it is clear that the current sociopolitical climate is not conducive to changes which imply increased government spending in the community services sector, or most other sectors (Sheil 1997, p.5). On the other hand, as the whole system of industrial relations in Australia proceeds apace along the road to enterprise based, individual agreements with a minimal role, or no role at all, for either trade unions or for a central arbiter or conciliator, the opportunity for carers to argue their case or exact concessions, fades inexorably. These so-called reforms are now well advanced. They were begun under a Labor regime and have simply been accelerated under the conservative Coalition Government (comprising the Liberal and National Parties). In these circumstances the call from a relatively small and, in some respects, marginalised group of women workers for consideration of their special circumstances is unlikely to be heard, let alone acted upon (Pocock 1995; Nightingale 1995).

The one hopeful sign in this general picture of gloom is the inclusion in the enterprise agreements which have been negotiated within a number of organisations and companies, of special "carer's leave" provisions. Our own university is one such organisation. This is a notable development but it must be remembered that leave provisions of this kind would once have been entrenched in legislation which imposed on all employers (or employers in workplaces over a specified size or in specified sectors) a legal obligation to institute these provisions. Some writers remain hopeful that the introduction of enterprise bargaining will expand family related workplace benefits providing "an area where negotiation for flexibility and family friendly policies could have considerable impact" (Edgar 1995, p.281). To date there is little evidence that this has been the case (ACIRT 1998).

The second issue of concern is of a rather different nature. This is the recognition of how little change, indeed how little real progress, has occurred in women's working lives, both in terms of their position in the paid workforce, and in the field of unpaid caring work. It is not just that caring has remained substantially a "gendered" activity, but that the double load that has been the almost universal experience of women entering the world of paid work, has remained so firmly in place. The rhetoric has changed. At this level there is a recognition that men must take a greater responsibility for domestic work and share the unpaid load (de Vaus 1997). The reality, however, the actual experience of women's lives, has changed little since the seventies, since the re-entry of married women to the labour market and the advent of second wave feminism and a broadly based women's movement. What has proved especially revealing is that the actual nature of the wife's labour market participation - casual, part-time or full-time - brings about only marginal increases in her male partner's unpaid work contribution. Being married, that is, having a male partner to "care for" and, most especially, having children, is what changes the woman's unpaid load. The care of frail elderly relatives is simply added to these existing responsibilities. In spite of the different family circumstances created by married women's full-time work commitments and in spite of the "New Age" rhetoric of equality and equal sharing of the unpaid load, women continue to undertake the bulk of the unpaid housework and the caring within the family and beyond (Baxter, 1993; Bittman 1992; Bittman & Lovejoy 1993; Bittman & Pixley 1997; Goodnow & Bower 1994; Ironmonger 1989).

In addition, the policies that have attempted to bring about fundamental changes in the workforce and in women's participation have not had the significant impact they were meant to have (Poiner & Wills 1991). There are said to be a number of factors at work. Some writers have argued that men continue to resist these changes and that the sexual division of labour, which has been particularly marked within the Australian workplace, has faded only marginally under pressure from these reforms or from the major restructuring of workplaces across the country. The sexual division of labour has simply been reaffirmed and taken new forms. The general pattern remains intact - "men and women continue to occupy different positions in the labour market, because of its high level of segregation, both horizontally (across industries and occupations) and vertically (within industries and occupations)" (Bryson 1995b, p. 65). Probert, drawing on Game and Pringle's 1983 study of gender relations in industries undergoing major technological change, argues that work is reconfigured in such ways as to maintain power relations and the differences between male and female spheres. She concludes, "It is quite possible for jobs to change their sex. What seems far less likely to happen is for jobs to lose their association with one particular sex, and to become 'gender-neutral' " (Probert 1997, p.324). In addition, the socialisation of women in the education system at all levels, including the subjects they most typically study and those they "avoid", has disadvantaged them in the competition for jobs, and the traditional cultures of most organisations and professions have not been particularly appealing to women.

All of these factors and more have made it difficult for the equal employment policies introduced by both State and Federal governments in Australia, to have the desired effect. The result has been a workplace environment that has changed far less than might have been predicted given the sheer impact of large numbers of women, especially married women, in paid work and given the major policy initiatives that sought to ensure more equitable female participation at all levels and in all sectors, more equitable remuneration that reflected this new participation and new ideas about women's work. The philosophy of equal opportunity has too frequently been interpreted as "a strategy to make girls more like boys, women more like men". The aim must be rather to promote "the idea that men should do domestic science and child care" (Ibid., p.325) and, we might add in this context, care of the sick, the disabled and the frail elderly.

There are two reasons for introducing an argument about equal employment policies in a study of this kind and at this point in the book. The first relates to our concern with the need to change workplace environments so that they become more attuned to the family and caring responsibilities of both men and women workers. What this brief discussion of workplace reform demonstrates is just how little change has actually occurred in Australian workplaces in response to increased female participation and to the policy interventions that have attempted to recognise the rights of working women. It also reveals how difficult it has proved to bring about change in this arena. Work environments tend to be neither responsive to women's claims for an equal share of the rewards of work (money, status and power), nor to the family responsibilities which women have typically borne. This would suggest that further attempts to address the needs of women, for example, to ensure a recognition of elder care and a palpable response to that recognition, are going to face similar opposition and "stonewalling".

Secondly, what we learn from an examination of equal opportunity policies and their application is the need for a radical re-think of the basic premises and assumed strategies of all policies in this area. If there is to be any chance of reform of the kind that our participants are calling for, then we need changes that attempt to make men and the male workplace more, dare we say it, "feminised". Some of the ways in which this might be achieved include campaigns to raise the status of "womens' jobs" and to re-value women's working skills. This latter strategy might be possible if attempted on a case-by-case basis as part of the re-structuring of industrial awards and individual workplace agreements (Ibid., p.326) but our own view is that the signs are not favourable.

In examining the need for workplaces to be radically reformed we are brought back to the need for a re-thinking both of what we define as the "ideal worker" and of what we think of as "normal work". We have already discussed at some length the notion of the ideal or model worker but have only referred briefly to the notion of normal work.

Belinda Probert has written about the need to bring about a "strategic focus on ways of making part-time work a normal aspect of working life, with as many training and promotion opportunities as full-time work". In making an argument for this kind of restructuring of normal work, she is at pains to underline the importance of ensuring that, in recognising that the "vast majority of women will continue to chose to combine paid and unpaid work", we do not fall into a way of addressing complex and, seemingly, intractable labour market problems which "yet again asks women to do all the adapting". Probert emphasises, as have many other feminist writers, that "(t)here is a very real danger that women will simply remain in part-time, low paid work, without careers, in order to preserve valued patterns of caring work" (Ibid., p. 327-8).

If giving part-time work status and security is one solution with benefits for carers in a range of different circumstances and of both genders, there are other reforms that should also be considered. In their exemplary book on contemporary families (and government provisions and state responsibility, and the labour market and employers), Bittman and Pixley refer to "the concept of 'time sovereignty' from Germany, where workers can structure their work day around their caring responsibilities" (1997, p. 266). Of even greater importance, they argue, is the need to reduce the number of hours which constitute the working day, itself. Instead of the current 50 to 70 hour week, which those in paid employment "enjoy", we need a reduction in what is expected or required of all workers. This, say Bittman and Pixley, "along with public provision of services, both creates more employment and reduces the cares and burdens of family life" (Ibid., p. 267).

We might summarise the changes needed in the workplace as being; change in the notion of the ideal worker, change in the notion of the normal job and change in the concept of the normal working day. This re-ordering of working hours and conditions is essential, but, as we have already stressed, it is a particularly difficult task in a workplace which is one of the least flexible and most sex-segmented in the developed world (Baxter et al. 1990; Munford 1989). Nor is it likely to come about without government intervention. Yet the notion of reshaping the market, even reshaping it in the interests of the family, is fundamentally at odds with the neoliberal construction of the appropriate role for governments. And it is a neoliberal philosophy that continues to hold sway in Australian political debate even if the edge of neoliberalism has been dulled in the United States and in Britain.

> *If neoliberalism is dying, just as obviously it is not yet dead, nor is the alternative future direction clearly discernible - at least not in Australia. Indeed, despite experiencing all of the globe's recent economic cycles, the political pattern in Australia (and New Zealand) has at least superficially stuck out in contradiction to the main world direction"* (Sheil 1997, p.3).

Recognition of elder care

This research highlights the need for the proper recognition of this increasingly significant area of family responsibility. From such a recognition flows all the other implications; without it no real reform is possible. What does recognition mean?

In the first instance there must be an acknowledgment that the demographic trends do in fact imply a greater chance that those in the workforce will find themselves with responsibility for providing a level of care for some elderly relative or friend for some period during their working lives. For most of these workers the time they will have to devote to a heavy caring demand will be limited. Most elderly people remain in good health through their latter years. When there is ill health or an accident resulting in injury, then the care required may be intense but is likely to be short term. In other instances it may be the case that there are longer periods of semi-care.

We cannot ignore the fact that the number and proportion of the frail elderly will increase and this does have implications for those with relatives in this category. Many of these potential carers will still be in the paid workforce and will want to remain working. Their own future security depends on it. The time when it could be assumed that the women of the family would be available to provide both short term and ongoing care are past. It is not reasonable to expect some workers and potential workers to forego work and security to provide intensive caring. This in no way denies the importance of family care nor takes from the devoted care that many provide, full-time or part-time, but we cannot premise our policies on this expectation.

Future projections of "caring-demand" which are based on co-resident caring alone will not reflect the real level of demand for care. This study, with its more wide ranging definition of a major caring responsibility, underlines this. If, in addition, we acknowledge the importance of both semi-care and "caring about", then the implications for the picture of "caring-demand" which we construct and the repercussions of this in the workplace, are profound. To claim that all workers who have relatives and friends who are elderly will find themselves with some level of responsibility for their care at some time, may not be an overstatement. Add to this demand the requirement to care for children, siblings and friends not yet elderly, and we have a picture of family demand that includes virtually all workers at some point in their careers. In Australia in 1993, 16% of carers who were in paid employment, often had need of time off work because of their caring responsibilities (ABS 1995). The consultant group, *Families at Work*, estimated that, on average, per annum, per employee, three days were lost and more than four days disrupted, due to problems with adult dependant care responsibilities (Department for Women 1997).

We cannot, however, treat the care of the elderly and the provision of child care in the same way. Recognition of this family responsibility means that the unpredictable and stressful nature of elder care must be recognised and the difference from child care fully appreciated. Whilst much has been written on this stress as it occurs in *mothers* in full-time employment, the specific difficulties of the stress for employees caring for older relatives has not often been examined in detail. These difficulties are numerous and our study has highlighted a number of them. They include:

* the less predictable demands of the dependent older person. (Unlike a child whose four year preschool period is predictably followed by the need for after school care.)

* the fact that the relative needing care has been an independent adult who cannot be ordered about. (Children do learn that their well being depends on fitting in with more powerful adults, at least to some extent.)

* the right of the relative to refuse formal services even though the carer can see that agreed standards of hygiene and safety are dropping. (With children the obligation to the child's future makes health and safety standards clearer, whereas with the notion of the ageing process ending inevitably in death, it is harder for a carer to insist on standards which may compromise the older person's less tangible quality of life issues.)

Recognition also means cataloguing the skills and personal qualities that caring work entails. These are not just the important nurturing, vicarious skills and capacities for patience, selflessness and altruism that we tend to associate with caring. There are, as well, skills in management of time and of competing demands, skills in dealing with people in difficult and often distressing circumstances. All the knowledge, competencies, capacities and skills that we have already documented here are of importance. Failure to acknowledge this wealth of wisdom and of what are often called "people skills" and failure to give real status to them in the workplace, is a loss on two counts. We miss out on using those skills in any particular instance but we also demonstrate again how little value we place, in any event, on certain kinds of skills and knowledge. The lack of valuing of these so-called "feminine" skills has been commented upon in many different contexts. What we want to emphasise here is the absurdity of this denial. This denial also represents a kind of hypocrisy in these days of multi-skilling. And it is hypocritical in another important respect because there is a sense in which we all know how important these things are to any kind of community not least of all to our workplaces.

Changing the nature of organisational culture

This suggests the need to re-examine the organisational cultures we have promoted in most workplaces. If we are to develop workplace environments that acknowledge and respect the family responsibilities of their employees, we are going to have to change the organisational cultures that operate within them. The places of work in which we sought most of our participants were the kinds of work environments in which, by their very nature, you might expect greater readiness to recognise the non-work obligations of employees. In some respects this was so and in a number of cases there was clear evidence of a high degree of recognition and support for the caring responsibilities of workers as mentioned above.

In most of these workplaces, however, as in work places generally, there was no real recognition of the "fact" of elder care and the strain it imposed on employees and certainly no provision for time off or a degree of flexibility in time of crisis. In some there was a clear message that there would be no allowances made and no special consideration should be expected.

Our research points to the need for workplace policies and organisational cultures which confer legitimacy upon the felt obligation and responsibility to care for older relatives which many workers already have and many more will come to have in the future.

This recognition of the skills learned in caring should also lead to a redefining of the ideal employee and employer so that they do not exclude full-time employees who temporarily or intermittently may have to give the care of an older relative priority over work. Rather, such persons should become greatly in demand as having already achieved, at no cost to the employer, urgently-needed people skills. These are currently taught at great expense to senior managers in work time.

Recognition of the importance of elder care, changed organisational cultures, redefinition of what a model worker "looks like", a valuing of the skills and knowledge that caring entails and the relevance of these to the world of paid work, all these changes are necessary and vital. They are needed not only for those who are caring now and not just for the sake of those who will find themselves in the future with some level of responsibility for the care of an elderly parent or other relative: but they are needed by us all, workers and employers alike. Such changes will create work environments that are better and happier places to work for everyone.

A few concluding comments

Caring is everyone's responsibility. This study calls for a proper recognition of caring and of what it entails on the part of all sectors - the community at large, the three levels of government, the community service sector, private welfare agencies and the workplace. We acknowledge that there is in all of these areas of the community some growing acceptance of the importance of caring activity and the work of carers. But that recognition is far from adequate.

More especially, we would argue that the workplace must change if workers with caring responsibilities are to be enabled to work and care. It is not just that the demographic changes that are already apparent will require that most people, and so most workers, will have a level of care for some period of their lives; nor is it just that for most of these workers, the time of greatest caring demands will be limited. What must be emphasised is that caring is not for ever and that most carers want and deserve the security of continuing work. These are important considerations but do not in themselves constitute the full picture nor the complete reason why workplaces must change.

If, as we argue, caring work is everyone's responsibility and all workers have family responsibilities, then we have got to completely revamp the values that attach to the ideal worker or manager and thus to what constitute legitimate adjustments of workplace routines, use of company time and facilities, and general conditions of work. We cannot value caring work, accept the premise that workers have family responsibilities and continue to operate with such a perverse, distorted and unnatural a conception of the ideal and serious worker.

There is, of course, a wider political and social context for all that we have discussed here and for any proposed changes that might be advocated. What emerges from this study and from others like it is a complex and disturbing picture which is comprised of a number of significant elements. These reflect the arenas in which the worker with caring responsibilities must operate - the caring role, the paid work force, the rest of the family, domestic work. As well there may be the demands of dependent children. All of these areas of life are under strain and while they may always have been areas of difficulty (at least at times) and while it may always have been hard to fit into our lives the numerous and competing demands of home and work, what we confront here is a new phenomenon. Each of these areas is now under additional and sustained pressure and some are under immense strain. Most of this pressure is connected in one way or another with changes in the conceptualisation of the role of government, on the one hand, and of our competitiveness in world markets, on the other. The consequences for all of us, and most particularly for carers, have been reduced funding to community services and thus fewer services, shortened hospital stays and longer waiting lists, reduced income and wages that do not keep pace with inflation or rises in the cost of living, greater job insecurity for ourselves and our children, longer hours at work to get the same job done, and increased work load with so-called multi-skilling and productivity claims. For most of us these represent a deterioration in our standard of living, in our conditions of work and, thus, in the quality of our lives.

At the same time there is growing pressure to cut government spending and lower personal income taxes still further. What has become the unquestioned framework (or strait-jacket) for all discussion of the role of government is one which posits the necessity of small government. This has meant that the only two positions which are debated are either, an argument for further reduction across the board (except perhaps in the areas of policing, defence and corrections), or, the argument that we have cut enough, let's halt at this point. No one, seemingly, is prepared to argue for *increased* government spending, least of all in the so-called welfare sector.

Two important points must be made here. The situation we have just described is one that affects us all and for most of us the impact has been a negative one. That would seem reason enough for us to be questioning with vigour the set of assumptions on which such policies are based. But here is also an issue of natural justice. These policies impact far more destructively on those who are most vulnerable. That is widely acknowledged. What is not so often recognised is that the vulnerable include not only care recipients but care givers, the very people who sustain the community's unpaid caring load, especially in relation to elder care. This is so not only of co-resident full-time carers but of carers who have managed to stay in the paid workforce. Both groups of carers may be said to be "paying their way", as the neoliberal economists require of us all. In fact, in large measure, they bear the costs on behalf of the rest of us. They pay for the privilege of caring. We benefit. To state the position crudely, they are saving the tax paying public vast sums of money. If they are not adequately supported, then, in all likelihood, further payment will be exacted from them; they will pay with their health as well.

This brings us to the second point. If we fail to make adequate provision for the on-going support of the elderly and their carers, we simply increase the demand on the public purse; finally carer as well as care recipient will require care and such care will normally be provided by government funded health services and, in the case of the elderly, in nursing homes.

Support for carers is not "welfare" but astute and compassionate investment. Why should this area of government expenditure be labelled "welfare" and the "plethora of outlays... made by different tiers of government in Australia which directly or indirectly increase the profitability of private sector firms", be seen as investment (Mitchell 1995, p. 12)? We need perhaps to view unpaid caring work as an industry and so as a significant site for government investment.

So we conclude with a call for the kind of recognition of unpaid caring work which acknowledges it for what it is - an arena of productive work which has value for us all. It not only saves governments money, a great deal of money, but it helps to create the kind of responsible, caring and compassionate community from which we all benefit.

Appendix

THE EXECUTIVE SUMMARY OF THE REPORT PRESENTED TO THE COMMONWEALTH DEPARTMENT OF EMPLOYMENT, EDUCATION AND TRAINING (1995)

Aims of the research

The overall aim of the research was to investigate the experience of women who are both working full-time (or near to full-time) in the paid workforce as well as carrying a major responsibility of care for an elderly relative or relatives. There were two general objectives. First, to investigate how the women balanced the demands of caring and paid work, how caring shaped and constrained the other areas of their lives, and the implications of this both in the immediate context of managing a stressful life day-by-day but also the likely impact in the longer term. Secondly, to examine the nature of the support they had received from family, community services and, most significantly, within the workplace.

The definition of "a major responsibility of care" which is adopted in this research moves beyond co-resident caring to include as well care for relatives who continued to live independently and those in hostels and nursing homes. Thus, the decision as what constitutes a major caring responsibility rested with the participants, themselves.

This is social policy research. It takes a particular view of the nature of social policy, one that focuses on the direct impact of all public policies on the welfare of citizens and which defines policy as inclusive of all arenas of policy development and implementation. The view of policy which clients and customers provide is thus a significant dimension of social policy.

Who participated

Forty one women participated in the study. Forty were included in the final sample. All were working full-time (or near to full-time) and while they were drawn from a range of occupations, the majority were working in the human services, health sector and in the teaching and academic professions. They worked at all levels from professional and managerial, to secretarial and domestic.

The accommodation arrangements of the care recipients varied and included most possibilities - hostel, nursing home, co-resident and independent living (whether living next door, relatively nearby or living at a distance).

The state of health and degrees of dependency of the elderly relatives also varied from those requiring intense and constant attention to those requiring general monitoring together with assistance when required.

The length of time the women had been responsible for caring varied form less than five years to thirty years.

How the stories were collected

Most participants were contacted through community service agencies and regional health systems, including hospitals.

The method of data collection employed was in-depth interviewing using a list of focus questions. Interviews were taped and transcribed for analysis.

The emphasis in interviews was on the experience of the carer and the particular meaning and value that each participant assigned to that experience. The extensive use in this report of quotations (some lengthy) from these interviews reflects this research approach.

Main themes and specific findings

The report begins with an extensive discussion of the experience of caring. Our participants made it clear that it was the experience of caring that absorbed most of their time and physical and emotional energy. Caring transforms the life of the carer and shaped all aspects of their lives.

The "choice" to care was rarely a straightforward or clear cut decision or, indeed a single "choice". Very frequently there were, in reality, few alternatives. The "choices" that were made reflected and were shaped by an ongoing, close and often complex relationship. Each caring situation had its own history which involved many "choices" and was influenced by many factors.

It was clear from the accounts that time spent caring was often more stressful and physically and emotionally demanding than paid work. A predominant theme was the emphasis on the emotional as well as the physical demands of caring. Some of the women spoke of their work as an escape from the pressures of caring.

Paid work was important to these women. For most it vital for their own financial security (immediate and longer term) and that of their families; it was also personally rewarding and a significant part of their identity.

Caring work was fitted around the demands of paid work. Work was the more predictable part of their lives. The need to organise and manage one's time as effectively as possible created tension and strain. Participants were, to a large extent, torn between work and family responsibilities and were constantly attempting to juggle the time and energy devoted to each. Most of the women attempted to keep the two spheres of their lives separate and tried to ensure family concerns did not intrude into the work context.

Nearly all the women had accepted restrictions and foregone opportunities for advancement in their work. Some had postponed or abandoned further education or had not sought promotion.

The need for understanding from employers, allied with a clear recognition that caring for an elderly relative is a legitimate activity, was a recurring theme. Some of the women had experienced severe difficulties negotiating time off during periods of crisis. Some employers were clearly unaware of the difficulties the women were facing. It would appear that the majority of employers did not see the caring circumstances of their employees as having anything to do with them.

All the women recommended increased flexibility in the way work is organised and wanted the opportunity to negotiate flexible working hours, vary work patterns and, perhaps, to be able to work from home, at least for periods when there was a crisis in the caring situation.

Most suggested a category of carer's leave be included in awards to enable them to apply for time off in a sanctioned and legitimate manner.

Arguments

Caring for elderly family members is an important and significant part of the family responsibilities that workers carry and needs to be recognised.

Those who work and care are carrying a considerable workload and receive inadequate recognition and support. The caring work they do represents significant cost savings to the government and their continuation in paid work for the time being and into the future, is some insurance that they will remain independent of state support, representing further potential savings. The "cost" is borne by the women themselves.

The number of people carrying some level of caring responsibility is likely to increase. Many of the carers will be in the workforce and will need, for their own financial security, to remain in their jobs. It is not reasonable to expect some workers to forego work and security to provide intensive caring. We cannot premise our policies on the expectation that the cost of such care be the future independence and security of the carer.

An overriding concern of the research is with how we change workplaces, government policy and community attitudes to create and foster a better and more supportive environment for workers who are caring, indeed for all workers and all carers.

The research points to the need to change workplace policies and organisational cultures to confer legitimacy on the felt obligation and responsibility to care for older relatives.

Recognition means recognising the skills that are acquired and developed through the experience of caring work. As well as the nurturing skills, capacity for patience and empathy, there are skills acquired in managing time and competing demands, skills in dealing with people in distressing and difficult circumstances. These skills are currently taught to senior managers in work time at considerable expense.

The categorical separation of work and family life is counter productive. There is a clear need to reassess this taken for granted notion and the concepts that flow from it, e.g., that of the ideal or model worker.

A number of critical concepts are re-examined. The study stresses the need to recognise the problematic nature of the "choice" to care and to avoid glib use of the term in policy debates. The concept of "time" and the different ways in which time is conceptualised and valued are also important in debates about caring although they receive little attention. Our understanding of "independence" is also discussed. The women in this study, although they have remained in the workforce and, in that sense, retained their independence, have, nevertheless, foregone "degrees of independence" as a result of their caring responsibilities. The report presents a typology of caring and argues for a recognition that almost all of us will, at some time in our working life, find ourselves with some level of caring responsibility even if for a relatively short period. It also proposes the need for a much more honest and fair-minded analysis of those factors and activities which waste time and decrease productivity in the workplace.

Finally, we call for a recognition that support for carers is an astute as well as a compassionate investment. Caring is an arena of productive work which has value for all of us.

References

Aronson, J. (1990), 'Women's Perspective on Informal Care of the Elderly: Public Ideology and Personal Experience of Giving and Receiving Care', *Ageing and Society*, vol. 10, pp. 61-84.

Australian Bureau of Statistics (ABS) (1996), *Focus on Families: Caring in Families Support for Persons who are Older or Have Disabilities*, Australian Bureau of Statistics, Catalogue No. 4423.0, Canberra.

Australian Centre for Industrial Relations Research & Training (1998), *Agreements Database and Monitor No. 16*, University of Sydney.

Baines, C.T., Evans, P.M. and Neysmith, S.M. (eds) (1991), *Women's Caring: Feminist Perspectives on Social Welfare*, McLelland and Stewart, Toronto.

Baxter, J., Gibson, D. and Lynch-Blosse, M. (1990), *Double Take. The Links Between Paid and Unpaid Work*, Australian Government Publishing Service, Canberra.

Baxter, J. (1993), *Work at Home: The Domestic Division of Labour*, University of Queensland Press, St. Lucia.

Bittman, M. (1992), *Juggling Time: How Australian Families Use Time,* AGPS, Canberra.

Bittman, M. and Lovejoy, F. (1993), 'Domestic Power: Negotiating an Unequal Division of Labour Within a Framework of Equality', *Australian and New Zealand Journal of Sociology*, vol. 29, pp. 302-21.

Bittman, M. and Pixley, J. (1997), *The Double Life of the Family: Myth, Hope and Experience*, Allen and Unwin, Sydney.

Bryson, L. (1992), *Welfare and the State. Who Benefits?*, Macmillan, Basingstoke, Hampshire.

Bryson, L. (1995a), 'Family, State, Market and Citizenship', in Weeks, W. and Wilson, J. (eds), *Issues Facing Australian Families. Human Services Respond*, (2nd edition), Longman, Melbourne.

Bryson, L. (1995b), 'Two Welfare States: One for Women, One for Men', in Edwards, A. and Magarey, S. (eds), *Women in a Restructuring Australia: Work and Welfare*, Allen and Unwin (in Association with the Academy of Social Sciences in Australia), Sydney.

Cass, B. (1993), 'Work and Family: The World Stage. The Work and Family Debate in Australia; Emerging Perspectives and Issues for Policy Debate in the International Year of the Family', *Work and Family: the Corporate Challenge*, Paper presented at AFC/BCA Conference, Melbourne, 1 December 1993.

Clare, R. and Tulpule, A. (1994), *Australia's Ageing Society*, Economic Planning Advisory Council, Background Paper No. 37, January 1994.

Cox, E. and Leonard, H. (1991), *From Ummm - to Aha!: Recognising Women's Skills*, AGPS, Canberra.

De Vaus, D. (1997), 'Family Values in the Nineties', *Family Matters*, Australian Institute of Family Studies, No. 48, pp. 5-10, Spring/Summer 1997.

Department of Health, Housing and Community Services (1991), *Aged Care Reform Strategy Mid-Term Review Report 1990-91*, Australian Government Publishing Service, Canberra, Australia.

Department of Health, Housing and Community Services (1991), *Aged Care Reform Strategy Mid-Term Review Discussion Papers 1990-91*, Australian Government Publishing Service, Canberra, Australia.

Department of Industrial Relations (1994), 'Work and Family Unit', *The Workplace Guide to Work and Family*, Australian Government Publishing Service, Canberra, Australia.

Department for Women and Families at Work (1997), *Aged Care, Facts for Australian Employers*, Sydney.

Disney, H. (1992), 'The Future for Community Services', *Impact*, vol. 22, No. 10, pp. 10-12, November 1992.

Edgar, D. (1992), 'Sharing the Caring. Rethinking Current Policies', *Family Matters*, No. 31, Australian Institute of Family Studies, pp. 40-55, April 1992.

Edgar, D. (1995), 'Sharing the Caring: Rethinking Current Policies', in Weeks, W. and Wilson, J. (eds), *Issues facing Australian Families: Human Services Respond*, Longman, Melbourne.

Freeland, J. (1997), 'The Anatomy of Vulnerability: The State of Unemployment in Australia', in Sheils, C. (ed), *Turning Point. The State of Australia*, Evatt Foundation, Allen and Unwin, Sydney.

Glezer, H. and Wolcott, I. (1997), 'Work and Family Values, Preferences and Practices', *Family Matters*, Australian Institute of Family Studies, No. 48, pp. 27-29, Spring/Summer 1997.

Goodnow, J. J. and Bower, J.M. (1994), *Men, Women and Household Work*, Oxford University Press, Melbourne.

Graham, H. (1983), 'Caring: a Labour of Love', in Janet Finch and Dulcie Groves (eds), *A Labour of Love: Women, Work and Caring*, Routledge and Kegan Paul, London.

Grieve, N. and Burns, A. (eds) (1994), *Australian Women: Contemporary Feminist Thought*, Oxford University Press, Melbourne.

Hicks, C. (1988), *Who Cares. Looking After Old People at Home*, Virago, London.

Howe, A. (1993) Personal Communication.

Ironmonger, D. (ed) (1989), *Household Work: Productive Activities, Women and Income in the Household Economy*, Allen and Unwin, Sydney.

Land, H. (1991), 'Time to Care', in Maclean, M. and Groves, D. (eds), *Women's Issues in Social Policy*, Routledge, London and New York.

Lewis, J. and Meredith, B. (1988), *Daughters Who Care*, Routledge, London and New York.

McDonald, P. (1993), 'Social Policy in Australia. The Family Dimension', *Family Matters*, Australian Institute of Family Studies, No. 34, pp. 44-46, May 1993.

McKinnon, A. L. and Odynak, D. (1991), *Elder Care, Employees, and Employers: Some Canadian Evidence*, A Discussion paper prepared for the Demographic Review Secretariat, Health and Welfare Canada, Population Research Laboratory, Department of Sociology, University of Alberta, Canada.

Mitchell, W. (1995), 'Business Welfare - a Legitimate Role for Government?', *Current Affairs Bulletin*, vol. 71, No. 6, April-May, 1995.

Mumford, K. (1989), *Women Working: Economics and Reality*, Allen and Unwin, Sydney.

Neal, M. B., Chapman, N. J., Ingersoll-Dayton, B. and Emlen, A. (1993), *Balancing Work and Caregiving for Children, Adults and Elderly*, Sage Publications, Newbury Park, London and New Delhi.

Nightingale, M. (1995), 'Women and a Flexible Workplace', in Edwards, A. and Magarey, S. (eds), *Women in a Restructuring Australia. Work and Welfare*, Allen and Unwin, in association with the Academy of Social Sciences in Australia, Sydney.

Onyx, J. and Maclean, M. (1995), 'Career Progression in the Community Sector', *Australian Journal of Social Issues*, vol. 30, No. 1, February 1995.

Parker, G. (1993), *With This Body. Caring and Disability in Marriage*, Open University Press, Buckingham and Philadelphia.

Pocock, B. (1995), 'Women's Work and Wages', in Edwards, A. and Magarey, S. (eds), *Women in a Restructuring Australia. Work and Welfare*, Allen and

Unwin, in association with the Academy of Social Sciences in Australia, Sydney.

Poiner, G. and Wills, S. (1991), *The Gifthorse: A Critical Look at Equal Employment Opportunity in Australia*, Allen and Unwin, Sydney.

Probert, B. (1993), 'From Overwork to More Work', *Impact*, vol. 23, No. 1, pp. 11-13, February 1993.

Probert, B. (1997), 'Women's Working Lives', in Kate Pritchard Hughes (ed), *Contemporary Australian Feminism 2*, (2nd edition), Longman, Melbourne.

Schofield, H. and Hermann, H. (1993), 'Characteristics of Carers in Victoria', *Family Matters*, No.34, pp. 21-26.

Sheil, C. (1997), 'Introduction', in Sheil, C. (ed), *Turning Point. The State of Australia*, Evatt Foundation, Allen and Unwin, Sydney.

Standing Committee on Community Affairs, February (1994), 'Inquiry into the Home and Community Care (HACC) Program', *HACC Options/Discussion Paper*, House of Representatives, Canberra, Australia.

Stehlik, D. (1993), *Untying the Knot: A Socialist-Feminist Analysis of the Social Construction of Care*, Centre for the Development of Human Resources, Edith Cowan University, Social Research and Development Monograph No. 7, Perth.

Vanden Heuvel, A. (1993), *When Roles Overlap: Workers With Family Responsibilities*, Australian Institute of Family Studies/Work and Family Unit, Department of Industrial Relations.

Watson, E. A. and Mears, J. (1989), *Women in the Middle; Care Givers with a Double Burden of Care*, University of Western Sydney, Macarthur, Sydney.

Wolcott, I. (1991), *Work and Family. Employers' Views*, Australian Institute of Family Studies, Monograph No. 11, Melbourne.

For Product Safety Concerns and Information please contact our EU representative GPSR@taylorandfrancis.com Taylor & Francis Verlag GmbH, Kaufingerstraße 24, 80331 München, Germany

Batch number: 10725923

Printed by Printforce, the Netherlands